Understanding Cystitis

Angela Kilmartin was born in 1941 at Brentwood, Essex, and was educated there at the Ursuline Convent. An attractive, slim blonde, she was a well-known figure in fashion modelling for six years until, having satisfied her ambitions in that field, she went into the acting and operatic world. After intensive full-time training and with exciting prospects already opening up professionally, she married Paul Kilmartin in 1966. Three days after her marriage cystitis began and recurred every three weeks for the next four years. With her marriage and her career in shreds, she turned to face this appalling enemy and, some six months after being told to pass water after intercourse, she founded the U and I club to teach prevention and management of cystitis to other women.

Acknowledged as the world's expert on self-help in cystitis, she leads a demanding life in London teaching, lecturing, writing and broadcasting both on radio and television. Her *Open Door* television programme won acclaim from the world's professional television personnel and brought in hundreds of thousands of inquiries. She has made a film called *Helping Yourself in Cystitis* and is following that with *Helping Yourself in Vaginal Thrush*.

Angela Kilmartin

Understanding cystitis

Text illustrations by Cynthia Clarke
Pan Books London and Sydney

First published 1973 by Heinemann Health Books
This edition published 1975 by Pan Books Ltd,
Cavaye Place, London SW10 9PG
ISBN 0 330 24495 7
© Angela Kilmartin 1973

Made and printed in Great Britain by
Richard Clay (The Chaucer Press) Ltd, Bungay, Suffolk

Contents

Foreword 7

Acknowledgements 8

Introduction 9

1 Cystitis 15

2 Some causes – not all 19

3 Some outcomes – social and medical 33

4 Some letters 40

5 The sexual organs 59

6 The renal organs 65

7 Stress 70

8 Children 73

9 Medical investigations 77

10 Medical treatment 92

11 Self-help 103

Summary 117

Glossary of terms 118

Index 121

To Chunky
who was well worth fighting for

Foreword

This book deals with a subject the doctors, on the whole, are not greatly interested in. And yet cystitis is probably one of the commonest illnesses of women. The reason for this medical disinterest is complex. To start with, the bladder, nestling down in the pelvis, tends to fall between several stools as far as specialist medicine is concerned. The gynaecologist is interested in the bladder when it slips out of position, as it does in a prolapse. The urologist gets excited about it if tumours or polyps develop, and of course the pathologist will always test the urine. But each of these sections of specialized medicine tends to love its glorious isolation. Togetherness is not a common medical trait, I'm afraid. And so the patient often gets left out in the cold to suffer.

But as long as there are people like Angela Kilmartin about they won't suffer in silence! And I only hope that, apart from generating a lot of patient interest, this very useful book will stimulate the medical profession too.

We, the doctors, don't know a whole lot about cystitis. Sometimes, in this condition, the urine appears to be sterile, and so instead of cystitis we talk of the urethral syndrome, when such patients get ill. Then there are women who should have cystitis, for they are passing infected urine, and yet they have no symptoms at all. Clearly fundamental research on a large scale is necessary before the problem of cystitis is really understood. In the meanwhile, *Understanding Cystitis* will really help many victims of this particular brand of medical nastiness.

January 1973
Eric Trimmer, MB, MRC, GP
Medical Editor, *Medical News Tribune*

Acknowledgements

My thanks are due to a host of people who, since January 1971, have supported my efforts to help both doctor and patient. By compiling a list I am so afraid that some might have escaped my memory that I have decided to make it a very short one, applicable only to the book itself:

Mr John Wickham, MS, FRCS, Consultant Urologist, Mr Desmond Bluett, FRCS, Consultant Gynaecologist, and Dr Eric Trimmer, who have been towers of encouragement and mines of medical information; Mrs H. Andersen for being such an efficient secretary and typist, and to the following doctors for so generously allowing me to use extracts from articles written by them especially for the U and I Club magazine – Dr Gordon Young, MD, BSC, DPH, Dr D. A. Leigh, Consultant Bacteriologist, and Mr D. Wallace, Consultant Urologist.

January 1973
AK

Introduction

To date this is the only book about cystitis aimed at the patient. Much has been written about it by doctors for doctors that is above the heads of the untrained, and, in truth, even above a great many of the trained. Only a very few devotees of Urinary Infection Research manage to wade through the very complicated literature at present available. So this book will, I hope, cheer and enlighten a great many people.

In 1966 I had a most promising career as an opera singer, coloratura to be more precise, with a high acting ability, having been trained in both subjects over a period of six years at the Guildhall School of Music and Drama, entirely on scholarships and awards.

In *July* 1966 I was one of the principal singers in the cast of *The Yeomen of the Guard*, performed during the Festival of the City of London at the Tower of London.

In *August* 1966 I was struck down with my first attack of cystitis three days after my wedding to a man I adored.

Over the next four and a half years I was to know utter heartbreak. In that heartbreak was a lost career, foundering marriage and a lost trust in God.

Out of that heartbreak came a fighting spirit, anger, insatiable curiosity about cystitis, also The U and I Club, Registered Charity No. 262946, founded to impart knowledge of Urinary Infections to both patient and doctor.

To date, this club has had some 14,000 women, men and children through its files, drawn mostly from the British Isles but also from thirty other countries. Press articles have gone out all over the world and U and I sufferers are to be found in India, China, New Guinea, Africa, America, Australia, Thailand and many other far-flung places. In 1974 inflation hit printing and ink prices so badly that the six magazines a year for £1.25 ceased and instead a new booklet has been introduced, copies of which can be obtained from the U and I club.

Whilst this Pan book is 'Understanding' of cystitis so the U and I club's booklet is entirely 'self-help'. Other booklets will be introduced on relating topics and some translations are already available again from the club's address.

The problem may be commoner than pregnancy and ranges over the globe knowing no particular racial, religious or geographical boundaries. Wherever there is a woman, there is cystitis. Four out of five women experience it at one time or another, and of these some have *recurrent* cystitis, be it once a month or once a year.

I remember the first chat I ever had with a fellow-sufferer. It was like an Archangel holding my hand and saying: 'There, there, dearie, I do understand, really I do!' The relief of being able to say 'urine' without a single qualm and knowing that she too had sat on a loo passing blood and screaming into a handkerchief to deaden the sound! We chatted for half an hour just like sisters although we had never known each other. She was a solid, sensible woman whose husband had left her because of her inability to have intercourse through recurrent cystitis, and at that time—four and a half years after my wedding day—I foresaw that her marital anguish could also become mine any day. On that same day when I had spoken to her, I had reached the very bottom of my own well of despair.

Six weeks previously I had had a urethral cauterization performed in hospital to prevent any further attacks of cystitis.

It was my third operation—the other two being investigations. Frigidity during intercourse had become the lot of both my husband and myself and it was with bated breath that we resumed sex after the cauterization. But there yet again two days later—on the day of that phone call—had come the familiar pain and incontinence together with a fear of future life and a hate for marriage that I just can only fail to describe —so I won't!

At 5am I was in my back garden thrusting my wedding dress and going-away outfit down into the depths of my dustbin and sobbing hopeless tears. Four years of young and loving marriage shoved into the baked bean and peach cans. Silence, too, had become a part of relationships between my husband and me, as it does I believe when marriage is in jeopardy, so he left that morning not knowing my heart was out in that dustbin and that I might not be at home, even to be silent, on his return from work.

As the attack abated slowly during the morning I rang every Urologist in the Yellow Pages until I found one who could see me that day in a last-ditch stand to save my sanity. As the Ss were reached, a Urologist gave me a 5pm appointment in Harley Street. At the end of examination and discussions he informed me that for one month I was to try passing water after intercourse. Expecting some modern scientific treatment I was wide-eyed and incredulous—almost unbelieving. But as I would know within the month whether the idea would work I might as well give it a try.

However, I still had to cope with a frigid husband, frightened of giving me any more pain, and this was another bitter pill. Despite these problems, the month went and no cystitis. With a little easing of the distress we reached the end of the third month free of pain, only to reach square one with another attack. To cut an untidy story short, it appeared eventually, after consulting a gynaecologist, that my hormone balance was upset, probably from all that I had been through, and that the vaginal epithelium (skin) was unhealthy. With a good dose of hormones it improved, and knowing now that attention to the two causes must be constant I live very happily in friendly and conjugal relationship with my husband to whose constancy and love I dedicate this book.

As for my career—it has vanished I think. My ambition now is never to let another woman in this country reach such sorrow from whatever cause her cystitis may stem—and there are many such causes. It is far more satisfying to alleviate pain and discomfort than to stand on a stage and receive a standing ovation—so I have discovered.

One young woman once wrote to me that she could not understand how cystitis as she knew it could possibly stop one from working, so long as there was a bathroom handy! I wrote back saying that as far as I was aware there was no bathroom in *The Magic Flute*! and that, whilst one may be able to shed a few tears of pain and frustration over a typewriter, one cannot sing a top F with blocked sinuses!

In 1973 I organized a survey amongst Club members. 750 out of 2000 women filled in their forms and the results speak not only of the misery of recurrent cystitis but also of the essential part which self-help plays in effecting relief of symptoms. Successful medical help—entirely lacking in these 750 women or they would not have joined my Club in the first place—is not the only factor in treatment. The patient *must* participate and the survey below shows just how effective the action can be in relieving the distress.

1 Have you ever had tranquillizers because of cystitis depression?   35% yes

2 Have you ever had to have psychiatric help because of cystitis depression?   6% yes

3 Has your home or career suffered because of cystitis?   68% yes

4 Have you had to leave a job because of cystitis?   16% yes

5 Has your marital relationship suffered in any way? 73% yes

6 Has your marriage been broken by cystitis? 2% broken, 3% at breaking point

7 How many times have you been admitted to hospital for:

(a) Cystoscopies 774

(b) Major renal surgery 50

8 Has the U and I Club cheered you up? 93% yes

9 Have the U and I Club's practical ideas helped at all? 89% yes

10 Has the U and I Club solved your cystitis problem? 18% yes

All answers are *direct* results of recurrent cystitis—no other factors are present.

I must say a word or two about the medical profession. As much education is needed here as elsewhere and the consultants who are now my allies are the first to admit this. I have only met with sympathy, help and encouragement from these men and women and my admiration for them in this very depressing, unglamorous and little-researched work is unbounded. Their clinics are overflowing, their time is limited and they make the best of modern ideas. I'd like to thank them very much for being such marvellous listeners and nice human beings.

Also I must thank the Press and Radio. Their reports and interviews, with just one stupid exception, have been honest and accurate both about cystitis and the Club. They have brought the attention of countless thousands to this vast medico-social problem and given to those who are in need the opportunity of realizing the existence of the Club's magazine.

To all those 'miscellaneous' people who do not fall into any particular category but who nevertheless have contributed in numerous ways to the success of the Club, I must say simply that you are all a part of its growth and history and you, too, have left your mark on its future success.

In heading the chapters that follow I just used thought

progression as a basic principle and fervently hope that by the end I shall have said all that I had intended to say. So, having given my reasons for this restless curiosity and the desire to see an end to the suffering of countless thousands, I shall begin.

1 Cystitis

Cystitis, which is a condition of the bladder, is not an illness, sickness, disease or infection standing alone. It is often combined with one or several other conditions.

Once this thought is well established in the mind life can become at least a little more mentally tolerable for the patient. As a consultant urologist puts it, 'It is an umbrella term for infections or unexplained bladder problems.' It is easier for the GP to say to the patient complaining of waterworks trouble that he or she has cystitis. It is a very official-sounding medical word and the patient goes away feeling satisfied that something has definitely been diagnosed with treatment by antibiotics indicating a quite serious ailment. The GP for his part knows his patient will recover from the attack through his 'modern' treatment and that his surgery time will be over all the faster for it. Both parties to the visit are satisfied and feel that each has also satisfied the other.

However, neither party has questioned what caused the attack—let's hope at least that they will with the first recurrence, whether it be in the near or far future.

Most inquiries show that this questioning seldom happens. One GP I know admitted that after the seventh attack he sends the patient for hospital tests and knows almost for sure that the patient will be back pretty quickly to him for another prescription. The final hospital test is generally a cystoscopy (I'll cover the question of examinations and tests in Chapter 9) when the surgeon can have a good look at the urethra and bladder through his instruments. Invariably this again shows nothing abnormal, although at least by this stage they have begun to look for a cause to explain the attacks.

If someone will only explain to the patient that a cause does exist somewhere and that, unless the patient co-operates fully with ideas to clue-up the doctor, he has a very long and arduous task ahead of him. So full patient/doctor discussion will pay dividends not only in time and money but also in a quick solution to the problem. It is also important that patients can feel free to consult anyone whom they would like to question about any aspect of their problem without having to fight their GP for this right.

'I'm not sure,' writes some prospective member, 'whether I do have what you call cystitis.' This again comes from the tendency of doctors to lump together different bladder and urethral problems under this lovely official-sounding word.

True cystitis has the following symptoms:

Pain
Increased frequency of urination, sometimes uncontrollable
Blood loss from the urethra whilst urinating

If any of my Club members still reach this stage I should be disappointed in them. No matter what the cause, this Club preaches the gospel of how to block the course of a full-scale attack and it is fully explained in the last chapter. It does not of course do anything at all to remove the cause.

For those of you who really want it spelled out—the cause is what you should be searching for, not alleviation of the resulting attack. Mentally this search lifts you above each attack so that whilst dealing with the attack as we recommend, your mind lifts above it and back to any reason why it started. By the time three hours are up you have made a great many notes and your attack is nearly over. You can then ideally visit your doctor to talk over your notes.

If, through ignorance, the attack goes on completely

unchecked then backache begins and temperature rises up to
104F, 105F. The patient goes into rigors—uncontrollable
shivering even though she is well covered. This is known as
pyelitis. It is dangerous. It means that the kidneys are now
involved in the 'infection' for infection it certainly is by now.
At this point someone will call a doctor, and then will come
antibiotics, bed rest and high liquid intake.

If this is allowed to happen too often kidney failure could
result eventually. Cystitis must never, ever be ignored. A
doctor must never, at any time, tell the patient he can do no
more for her, and a patient must never upbraid a doctor for
being unhelpful—no one can know everything! Besides, as I
shall point out, it is just as much within the patient's power to
effect a 'cure' as it is within the doctor's.

Cystitis can occur at any time, in any place, as recurrent
sufferers know only too well. Once it has begun there is
nothing for it but to retire to the nearest privacy and deal with
it. It will not go away or even get worse slowly so that you can
finish your outing! In most people bleeding begins within
$2\frac{1}{2}$ hours and the pain, of course, is intense. With a recurrent
sufferer whose urethral skin has been frequently damaged by
the ailment, the attack precipitates much faster. So again we
have another good reason why that patient/doctor discussion
must begin earnestly at the first recurrence.

The pain is a progressive one starting at any damaged point
in the urethra and ascending to the bladder. It ascends a short
step at a time so each visit to the lavatory is a mental problem
as well as a physical one. With the ignorant sufferer who has
not immediately begun a swift intake of bland liquids the
urine will be passed much more quickly than the kidneys can
manufacture it, resulting in short, highly painful acts of
urination. The urine is also highly concentrated and acidic
and this acts as a knife which opens up a little more of the
damaged urethral skin each time it flows over the area. On this

inevitable course the whole urethra soon becomes uncontrollable and the muscles at the top of it which allow the bladder to open and expel the urine soon become badly damaged, resulting in incontinence for the duration of the attack. Eventually one sits on the lavatory permanently or wraps a towel around the trunk like a nappy in bed, although hardly any urine comes out at all. Once the bleeding is well advanced the bloodstream absorbs some of the germs which have hitherto been isolated in the urethra and bladder, so that the whole body feels unwell and shivery.

You may remark that I have mentioned it only progresses thus far out of ignorance. I do not mean an uneducated person with little intelligence, I mean anybody at all who has not been informed of how to deal with an attack, be she labourer or director. At the most a doctor may mutter about drinking lots of liquid but why or how much is never discussed. A set of rules is called for to help the patient. The U and I Club has just this but, of course, not everyone belongs to it. In every GP's surgery there should be such a list freely available to each urinary patient, and we might one day accomplish it if pressure on the profession can be made strong enough.

But let me make it clear that that list of helpful advice on how to deal with the attack is in no way a substitute for the doctor's advice.

I am convinced that the main reason why cystitis is an apparent mystery to both patients and doctors is because they concentrate on treating the attack instead of searching with integrity for its cause.

Readers interested in joining the U and I Club should write to Ms Angela Kilmartin at the address given on page 111 or c/o Pan Books Ltd, Cavaye Place, London SW10 9PG, enclosing a stamped, addressed envelope.

2 Some causes—not all

There are two main avenues of exploration for your cause or even causes. They are never straight but intermingle because they meet at one end and the central reservation is very narrow. These avenues are the renal organs and the sexual organs, and each has a later chapter to itself.

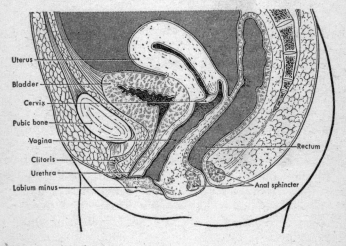

Uterus and vagina

As cystitis is predominantly a woman's ailment we shall disregard the male except where he, as the sexual partner, is involved in the female's cause.

Woman is susceptible to ascending infections because the

basic problem is one of bad architecture. She has in her perineum three openings all conducive to germ breeding and to bruising of the delicate tissues. Two of these orifices, the urethral and vaginal, are so close that they do in fact share the outer entrance and only separate when inside. The orifices are invariably and naturally damp with the mucous secretions able to contain a variety of organisms. The third one, the rectal orifice, is set further back and harbours inside a great many organisms harmful when out of their natural environment and unchecked by effective hygiene.

Cystitis results either from infection or bruising. The infection can either be of an ascending or descending nature in relation to the bladder—in other words it can already be present in the kidneys and bloodstream—or it can ascend from the perineum and urethra. Bruising generally results from sexual contact and, although it appears initially to present the same symptoms as infection, it is really only a reddening and swelling of the tissues which may afterwards begin to harbour organisms.

Let us discuss, firstly, cystitis in relation to the sexual organs and divide it into sexual activity and non-sexual activity.

SEXUAL ACTIVITY

The cause of the woman's cystitis can equally arise from the man as from herself, and only by discussing frankly their sex life as it began and progressed can the answer be realistic.

For instance, the old 'bride's disease' or 'honeymoon disease', etc, begins obviously in the earliest days of the sex life. The first question to be asked of both partners is, 'How was your sex life before your marriage?' If satisfactory answers result then one must assume that the problem has indeed begun during the honeymoon. From here one's mind questions mainly the aspect of regular and frequent honeymoon intercourse causing bruising and trauma. In other words, the sexual organs have been given little time between sexual sessions to recover their natural secretions and to have a simple rest. Athletes would not run two important races in one day. Neither would any kind of sportsman or woman subject their bodies to the strains and stresses of two competitions in twenty-four hours. Why should we expect these delicate sexual tissues to be different from legs and arms? They need to be thoroughly understood and respected.

On a honeymoon it might seem a little unromantic to wash before and after intercourse–too medicinal–so one carries on with the one-shower or bath-a-day routine. From the bruising standpoint this isn't enough, let alone the germ problem. Any inflamed area of your body is better off for a good rinse in cold water and the same goes for the sexual organs.

The main germ which causes trouble during and after sexual intercourse is one medically termed Escherichia Coli– E-coli to you and me. This lives in the bowel where it multiplies and dies quite passively whilst contained therein. But once out of this happy culture ground it is in trouble unless it can find another suitable breeding ground. Such a one is in normal acidic urine. So it must be stopped from reaching the main vaginal/urethral orifices. Underwear and hygiene enter this problem as can be imagined, and it is also here that this problem of bad female architecture comes in. A man's rectum is set far away from the danger ground of the tip of the penis, but a woman's rectum is one inch away from the main orifice with no effective barriers to the germs' progress up that inch beyond her own hygiene.

One other problem about E-coli is that it multiplies very, very quickly. In fact it multiplies by itself every 12·5 minutes. So if you have ignored your hygiene and ten germs find their way into your bladder then in 12·5 minutes' time you will have 10 × 10 = 100, and so on until tissue damage begins. This germ is especially violent in the act of intercourse. Spontaneous idealistic intercourse never thinks of hygiene and germs—a compromise must be worked out somehow by the couple beforehand. The thrusting movements in intercourse are also impressed on to the vagina's next-door neighbour—the urethra. Any germs lying around these two orifices will be pushed into the two openings and thus journey up and in with each thrust. As we know E-coli only needs a few minutes to multiply by itself, and if the wall of the delicate urethra has been slightly bruised during intercourse trouble is really in store. Well, you might say, why doesn't every married woman get cystitis? What makes some women get it and not others? We don't really know the answer, I'm afraid. Various theories are put forward such as the differing amounts of E-coli in individual bowels or the presence of individually higher levels of antibodies acting against it, or skin sensitivity.

There is no doubt that E-coli is responsible for a vast amount of cystitis.

As previously mentioned, the male partner has a stake, too, in cystitis relating to sexual activity. Apart from E-coli there are other groups of organisms which can 'ping-pong' between the sexual partners. Such a group is that of the trichomonas. It can easily be treated once identified.

Yet another is that of 'thrush'. Thrush also provides a good breeding ground for E-coli and depletes the natural vaginal secretions. It is a fungus-type of organism and a very tough, resistant one. Again it may be a common ingredient of the composite body becoming a problem only when the natural bacterial aids or flora have been cleared out by bad health or by other adverse conditions. Antibiotics are renowned for this action. They not only clear up infections but they also may remove the natural body resistants leaving a no-man's-land for the first invader to conquer–this often being Thrush.

Logically one can therefore say that the use of antibiotics can prolong or even cause cystitis.

An uncircumcised male presents a very great hygiene problem. It is difficult to cleanse thoroughly the foreskin which can harbour a multiplicity of bacteria. When intercourse takes place these germs are introduced into the female.

If intercourse is undertaken when the female is too dry, not only can bruising occur, but also cracking of the taut vaginal epithelium (skin or tissue), and bacteria can breed more quickly in a medium of blood, no matter how small the amount.

A full bladder enables bruising to occur more easily, as does a full bowel. They both provide walls of pressure during intercourse. Following on from this, certain sexual positions and hand-petting can again bruise or cause small lesions in the skin tissue.

There should thus be no doubt that the act of intercourse and its accompaniments can precipitate and cause cystitis. There is absolutely no reason why, with competent investigations by a GP or gynaecologist and all relevant swabs and tests plus patient self-help, many of these conditions should not be completely prevented and cleared.

NON-SEXUAL ACTIVITY

This section of causes presents more intricate problems and account must be taken of each woman and her anatomical individuality. Some main rules apply, but the possibility of diversity and adaptation must be readily recognized and accepted by the gynaecologist in charge of the case.

High up on the list we find hormones. A hormone, as my old biology mistress once described it, is a 'chemical messenger taking instructions from one part of the body to another'. I have since learned that there are scores of these messengers rushing around and really it's marvellous that ninety per cent of the time most of them work properly! But that odd ten per cent not in healthy working order is quite enough to mess up the messages so that 'B' doesn't get a clear instruction from 'A'. We still don't understand very much at all about these hormones. We know something about the more obvious ones that control conception and fertility, and about the ones controlling our output of urine, but there is a lot more to learn even about these.

One of the main reasons why hormones go astray is emotional stress. Stress stems from joy such as initial passion in sex, or sorrow upon the closing of a relationship. Stress acts upon the pituitary gland, situated at the base of the skull. The relevant messenger called gonadotrophin travels in the bloodstream to the ovaries telling them to release their eggs during ovulation in each menstrual cycle. Accordingly the bleeding ten days later is either slight or heavy, as is the build-up to it. Tenseness, irritability, irritation, water retention leading to weight gain, tender breasts and sometimes acute changes in the vaginal epithelium lead to a higher sugar level with a change of the acid/alkaline epithelial balance. Thus, back at the patient's level, we have an unhealthy vagina! The mucus in the vagina inevitably sticks around the orifice and begins to contaminate the vulva and perineum, also bringing the urethra into the picture. No amount of hygiene will prevent the spread of the infection.

Now, for a long while specialists have used either oral pills or locally administered creams to the woman experiencing cystitis during the menopause or after a hysterectomy. What the vast majority of specialists fail to realize is that women everywhere and of all ages from eighteen to eighty are liable to hormone imbalance, and not necessarily for any accountable stress situation. Hormone imbalance occurs when the normal male/female hormone balance is thrown out of gear and there is a lack of either or indeed both in the sexual system. Thus married or single girls and women are suspect all through their life-cycles and not just at the menopause. I believe that this accounts for a major cause of unexplained, recurrent cystitis and at time of writing there are a few research projects in further exploration of this known fact.

Contraception can start up cystitis in the previously non-troubled patient. In this case it becomes readily apparent that a complete unembarrassed honesty is necessary to root out the cause.

Various contraceptives are conducive to cystitis. The old-fashioned cap can cause simple pressure upon the bladder wall making the urge to void more frequent. Foams and jellies are very individual in their effect. For instance there is one particular vaginal foam contraceptive which has been proved culprit in many a case of 'stinging' or 'irritation', not just for the woman but also for the man having intercourse with her and I have heard several tales both medical and lay of this foam. By way of interest, this was the contraceptive that my husband and I took on our honeymoon but when I did eventually stop using it I still continued my attacks of cystitis despite the six-month period that doctors recommend to recover from this sort of experience. It has been known that despite cessation of chemical foams, the symptoms can persist for several months until the inflammation disappears.

Until suitable lubricants came along for general public use, women who had dry vaginas, be it for any reason, were often classed as 'frigid'. Nowadays a woman can reach to her bedside table for help. As a marriage progresses a woman just is not able to behave as she did in her courtship, honeymoon or early marriage, no matter how much she loves her man. Being in love is very different from loving and the successful marriage should contain both even if a lubricant takes over sometimes!

There is one well recognized lubricant, KY Jelly made by Johnson & Johnson. It is colourless, thin in substance and contains no therapeutic qualities. It is this lubricant which is mainly used by gynaecologists during vaginal examinations and it is also best for the cystitis patient.

To some women the contraceptive pill may have a causative effect, to others, it may mean remission of their symptoms.

Now from the word go, it is vital, I believe, that a fortnightly check of the patient should be made for the first two months, a monthly check for another four months and three-monthly checks thereafter. Also that most women should use a low-dose formulated pill. If after the third month the patient is still getting symptoms such as she may have experienced in the first, that particular pill should be stopped. But I do feel that diuretic help in the form of tablets should sometimes be given to aid the success of the pill. Very little can be done to ease the vagina as it readjusts to the new level of hormones (you will realize that the pill is in fact just hormones) beyond making sure that no thrush or trichomonal infections are present.

The main object of the pill is to inhibit ovulation, which is why, in the young woman, a three-year limit to pill-taking is recommended followed by a period of abstention.

I have mentioned the readjustment of the vagina to the possible higher hormone level in the blood. With the constant monthly and yearly prevention of this ovulatory process the ovaries are kidded into believing they are too old to work. The uterus therefore sheds very little blood and the vagina becomes drier and less elastic, giving an increased chance of infections.

However, during the first few months of readjustment to higher levels of oestrogen the vagina can become very moist with copious secretions. Thus ascending organisms may find successful breeding grounds either inside the vagina or at the orifice.

The pill-taking woman must be carefully supervised and any urinary problems should be reported. If the pill is suitable for the individual and weight gain is eventually negligible with no other troublesome side effect then during each three-year period the woman should feel very well indeed.

The small blood loss each month means that there is more and stronger blood circulating in the system, possibly providing a higher level of antibodies to fight invading bacteria. It is possible that urinary infections may be definitely eased if the pill suits a woman, but those first three months of trial may be difficult.

CHILDBIRTH

The uterus is a rather special female organ because in its cavity a new generation develops. It also can cause a woman to feel very off-colour if it is not properly cared for and respected. It is held in place by special bands of ligaments and muscles which support the growing baby for the nine months' pregnancy. If the uterus is to remain 'fresh' then its surrounding ligaments also must be helped to maintain their strength. Long periods of standing over the years or frequent pregnancies can cause terrific strain on these supports. Anaemia will prevent good strong blood from feeding these muscles and tiredness in general will make a woman lazy about 'holding herself in'! The eventual result may be a prolapse. A prolapsed uterus means that a section of the supporting tissue has failed and the uterus has 'flopped' down into the vagina. Degrees of severity vary according to how long the problem has been allowed to progress. Sometimes therapeutic exercises are enough but the worse the prolapse, the more likelihood there is of an operation to repair it. Prolapse does of course result in strain at some point on the bladder wall and this can bring about inflammation and frequency. So now you can understand why I have dwelt a little on the subject.

Pregnancy predisposes to chronic urinary infections in some women and completely clears up for the duration of the pregnancy in others! It's odd! Let us term the former Group A and the latter Group B.

Group A can count amongst their individual cases quite a large proportion of women who undergo a 'gear change' in their urinary motor! In other words our friend the supporting muscle doesn't work quite so efficiently because (a) he's stretched and (b) he's more than likely got a baby's foot inhibiting his movements! Consequently the urinary muscles become sluggish and the urine doesn't flow out so quickly—it comes out, but only slowly and there is always the chance that the odd drop is left out of the main downward flow somewhere to get stale and lead to blood-borne infections. Certain changes take place in the ureters which become very soft and bloated, allowing fine droplets of urine to linger. Hormones also are thought to account for the 'gear change' but research is still in progress here.

Group B, under which category I myself was placed, can really only be accounted for by the hormonal change which prevents the uterus from shedding its monthly lining of blood, as with the contraceptive pill which has the same effect. It is entirely an individual affair depending on whether your hormones were balanced or not before your pregnancy. Mine were not, so possibly they became balanced with the extra pregnancy hormones!

So much for cystitis with a sexual background. Now for a few renal problems—only a few main ones because really they are very numerous and again, like the problems relating to sexual organs, extremely diverse in their variations.

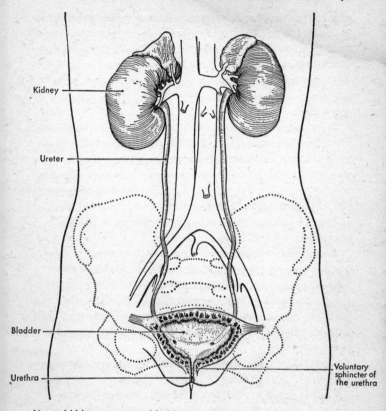

Normal kidneys, ureters, bladder, urethra

The renal organs comprise (as we will discuss at length later) the kidneys, ureters, bladder and urethra, and we are still discussing causes of urinary infection.

Let us start from birth. As with other parts of the body it is quite possible for congenital deformities or abnormalities to occur in the renal organs. One of the most common of these conditions is something called a refluxing ureter. It is mostly a childhood ailment and is due to faulty valve mechanism at the top bladder opening. The downward-flowing urine is squirted back again up the ureter towards the kidney because the faulty valve closes before all the urine has passed through into the bladder. Once back inside the ureter it tends to get a little stale and doesn't need much help to harbour offending organisms.

If the infection is not successfully contained and eliminated, the kidneys become involved and consequently damaged. So if the trouble continues beyond the age of eight years, when stronger muscle growth gives the faulty valve more strength to work correctly, then an operation is usually recommended. This refluxing ureter gives trouble in the bladder and urethra of course, with the odd infected patch of urine depositing germs as it flows through.

Ascending infections in childhood are also possible if the bladder is never emptied completely by the energetic child who is bored by the act of micturition and wants to pursue his or her interests uninterrupted! Also by the child who 'holds it' rather than ask to leave the classroom! Again E-coli from the rectum is the main culprit if hygiene is not regular and competent.

Later on in life diabetes accounts for a proportion of urinary discomfort and there is also a condition known as pre-diabetes. The latter is by name not so severe in its outcome as actual diabetes. The trouble is caused by excess sugar in the bloodstream and subsequently in the urine. The glucose acts as a food for E-coli in which medium it multiplies beautifully! So the diabetic numbers amongst his or her symptoms fairly regular attacks of cystitis.

A diverticulum is the growth on the bladder wall of another tiny bladder. You know sometimes you find a potato with another tiny one growing on it? Well it looks like that, except that there is a hollow tube connecting the two. Through this tube passes urine from the main bladder into the secondary one where, unfortunately, it gets trapped and cannot be drained properly. Thus it becomes stale and conducive to bacteria which eventually breed there.

A similar kind of state occurs in obstruction by kidney stones. Obstructions are termed loosely as any blockage interrupting the complete flow of urine from the kidneys to the bladder and thence out by way of the urethra. There may be a growth of excess tissue or cysts at any point along the renal channels, perhaps at the junction of the kidney and its ureter; a thickened bladder wall which limits the amount of urine able to be stored in the bladder space; something called, medically, trabeculation of the bladder, which to you and me is a roughening of the bladder lining enabling it to harbour germs (look at a map of the Norwegian coastline and you'll see what I mean!); almost anything that blocks the passage of urine.

A stone constitutes an obvious blockage, but the fact that it can be a moving blockage and very, very painful too puts it in a class by itself.

Catheterization of the urethra by instruments is also a known cause of implantation of bacteria into the bladder. Even in the best hospitals sterility of instruments can sometimes be suspect, and indeed if not handled with great gentleness once inserted, they can cause friction or cracking of the delicate tissue.

Herpes – the cold-sore virus – can also be present in the prostatic tissues of the male and be passed either by mouth or normal intercourse into the urinary organs of the female, although it can start in the female just as easily off its own bat. However, such research as has been done into connecting the herpes virus with chronic kidney infections has so far been unsuccessful.

Briefly to list a few other causes associated with urinary

infection we find nephritis, renal sclerosis, infections of the kidneys, hydronephrosis, calculi of the kidney and ureter, urethritis, stricture of the urethra, orchitis and epididymitis! Take your choice!

3 Some outcomes—social and medical

Cystitis is considered by specialists to be a great medico-social problem. The recurrent sufferer not only creates a strain within the family but presents a time-consuming problem to the medical facilities of our country.

Perhaps I might speak from personal experience of the two sides. Firstly, despite a costly honeymoon abroad, my husband and I had no proper relationship after the third day. We might as well have been on a single-with-parents holiday. The one revered and memorable holiday which young lovers can ever have was utterly ruined for us and we are by no means the only ones. Why didn't anyone tell me about the after-effects of intercourse? Pregnancy I knew about and VD didn't enter the arena at all, but what of the extra hygiene processes? Whose job is it to tell a young bride these things? No one ever does and I do believe that the only women equipped to begin a marriage are nurses who learn these things in the more dispassionate atmosphere of training. Although even in this profession it is possible just to miss out on the relevant lecture for reasons of illness, etc.

If this book does no other good than to make a few more honeymoons as enjoyable as they should be for memories' sake, then it will have achieved a lot.

From our honeymoon onwards a set of circumstances, seemingly beyond our control, for five years made a laughing-stock of our marriage vows. But ours only lasted the five years—what about the couple who, after thirty-two years of marriage, were finally helped decisively to have a reasonable sex life? The husband was so thrilled that he went home for lunch and sex every day to make up for all those previous heartbreaking years. Thirty-two years! The trouble is that they are not unusual, as doctors can testify.

All right, so honeymoons can go wrong for all sorts of reasons, but when one particular reason keeps on coming back at most unwanted and unexpected times with no hope of it ever ceasing, then that hitherto purely physical distress can become a mental distress as well. It is no secret that many recurrent sufferers from this ailment need psychiatric help, and it is also known that any specialist researching the problem and in close contact with each patient guinea-pig is prone to eventual depression himself.

My husband and I took six months to re-acclimatize properly to a balanced marriage after all that we had been through and the sexual side remained disjointed for an even longer period once back on the main road.

Within those five years of marriage came evenings of bitterness, hate and silence. Evenings when I vacated our double bed for the spare bed, others when even the six-foot width of our bed was just not enough. It became obvious to our friends and relations that each other's taunts were definitely aimed to hurt and that a gulf had opened up between us. Comments were made and the occasions of my public tears were becoming frequent. For each of the five years we took some sort of holiday, either at home or abroad, and each one was fraught with pain, embarrassment and depression. To mention an incident on our honeymoon—I was incontinent for a period of something like four days before I saw a doctor, and afterwards because the infection had taken such a hold. During that latter time I was given a urinary antiseptic pill which contained a blue dye. The floors of our honeymoon hotel were white marble. One evening I couldn't turn the key in the lock of our bedroom door quickly enough and the horror as I looked at the blue stain spreading over the marble will remain in my mind till I die.

What sort of memory is this of a honeymoon? And yet all I needed was a homely chat or a dispassionate discussion on hygiene. Three years on into our marriage, after one of my operations, a doctor muttered something about stepping up my hygiene—at that moment I nearly hit him—I was bathing every day—what more could I do? But since then, of course, I realize that the only way in which he offended was by his absence of any further discussion of it. I needed it spelt out to me, as everyone does who has received no medical training.

Alongside my failing marriage was running my failing career. If one has been up since 3am crying, drinking large amounts of water, taking a lot of painkillers and spending a depressing amount of time in the lavatory, one is in absolutely no shape mentally or physically to start singing love songs or death songs or glory to God! They just don't ring true! Many is the time I have collapsed in a flood of tears whilst singing extracts from *The Creation* by Haydn. There is a small section of recitative sung by Eve to Adam: 'Oh thou for whom I am, my help, my shield, my all. Thy will is law to me so God our Lord ordains, and from obedience grows my pride and happiness'. This always ended with me flinging the wretched score as far as I could!

Even if one managed to get the voice in trim, who on this earth would employ a singer likely to step down at any time through incontinence. Being a sensible person, I took my thoughts back to why everything was going so wrong. The answer was a physical ailment, and until it was cured or prevented I stood no chance of achieving a decent marriage or successful career. Then I dropped everything and set out upon a full-time search for help.

Previously I had run the gamut of fourteen types of antibiotics and various doses of each of them. I had urine tests,

X-rays and discussions with my GP and referral specialists, all on the National Health Service. When it dawned that the NHS was stumped for a solution I used my BUPA registration for private treatment. Under their auspices my husband and I used up something in the region of £2,000 with private tests, swabs, X-rays, cultures and three operations. None of this succeeded either! By this time despair was apparent in my walk, my features, my language and my attitude, plus thorough disillusionment with doctors everywhere. Just what paths could I tread next? The third operation had failed, and when that was readily apparent I abandoned all 'legal' methods of obtaining medical advice. I bluffed my way into the consulting rooms of the first specialist in urology who could see me on that dreadful day and by a miracle this was the man to begin parting these thick curtains of ignorance. Thus my long, slow and still painful recovery began—it was to be eighteen months later that the problems were completely overcome and, although I shall be prone to cystitis all my days, I can at least understand and prevent my own personal causes with a little medical help.

But what a waste of two young lives, what a waste of my talents and ratepayers' monies, what a waste of all that medical money and time, when all I needed was some simple homely advice! And I stress again that I have been lucky!

I think into the category of this chapter comes the U and I Club, Registered Charity No. 262946. It is an outcome, and one of the happier ones, of cystitis. Advice and cheer is now available for those who feel bereft. It is hailed by specialists as one of the most important advances in this field of medicine for many years and is frequently mentioned in lectures and discussions both on radio, TV and the press. Its main aim is to make the patient and doctor get together to solve the individual's cause, because above all else we want the sufferer to get better. The incidental aims like medical student grants and research subsidies come in a secondary category and will continue in future years, but each patient only has the one life and it is important that they are helped to enjoy this life. Our booklet is now available from the U and I Club and is chatty, humorous and practical in its writings. However, as previously explained, this book it is hoped will appeal just as much if not more.

My story is just one of a multitude; others follow through with separations, divorces, tremendous emotional upheavals, acute depressions, psychiatric treatment, and not at all unknown are threatened and successful suicides.

Children have a special problem because the rigours of school routine and running the gauntlet of schoolmates' taunts take a lot of courage to face if the child is unwell.

Leaving the classroom frequently is an embarrassment and trying to concentrate on work as well as trying to 'hold it' just cannot be done. Undoubtedly their education is impaired with so much time away, and the child's young world consists of scaring experiences on a doctor's couch. It must be very difficult to make and maintain friendships under such circumstances and, although I do not speak from any personal experience, I can well envisage it. My accuracy of imagination was verified one evening at a reception that the U and I Club gave. One of the friends of a guest had been nodding agreement all through the part of my speech relating to children and afterwards she spoke with tears in her eyes telling me how much she had suffered in her childhood and that I was absolutely correct in my points. Funnily enough she hadn't known until her arrival who or what our reception was about!

In these days time costs money. This being true I dread to think what this nation spends on urinary infection each year. The items on the bill are as follows: cost of drugs, creams and mixtures; GPs' time; urine cultures; swabs; X-rays and cystoscopies; general hospital and theatre staff; and all of these not just once but many times for *each* patient! When all of these have failed to provide knowledge of the cause then we follow on with psychosomatic or psychiatric treatment. Heaven only knows the prices because they are not the same two years running these days!

Whenever Fleet Street columnists write about cystitis and the U and I Club one of the first things they do is to walk round their office questioning the girls and women about it. Without fail affirmative statements are forthcoming.

When I first approached a city teaching hospital about starting our Club's magazine the Senior Urologist there invited me to meet all his associates and staff on a Friday afternoon. Everyone was called in—nursing staff, registrar, professor and technicians together with consultants, and we all agreed without reservation that everybody would be helped considerably if the patients would help themselves a little more. The numbers were so great seeking help from the clinics at the hospital that the doctors were pleased to be assisted by a lay woman on the aspect of patient self-help.

One is forced to wonder why these clinics are overflowing! To speak plainly there are two reasons:

1 Unclean and ignorant patients (lower, middle and upper classes)
2 Many irresponsible or ignorant GPs.

The modern GP is very fond of his antibiotic treatments. Telling a woman to wash more frequently each day seems a little absurd so they don't bother. Patients put themselves in the hands of their GP and in many ways even today they never discuss openly what is in their minds. If their cystitis occurs before a period or after intercourse they must say so. It is as much the patients' job to get themselves better as their GP's, and if the two of them got together in calm objective discussion a little more often a noticeable improvement might be seen in the numbers of hospital cases. I also feel that IVP X-rays and cystoscopies should not prove necessary for many patients, likewise the urine cultures in profusion. One thorough urine test should be all that is needed to ascertain whether cancer, glucose or other such harmful indicative organisms are present. E-coli bacteria infections should not prove problematical.

If some of these utterances were to be noted an awful lot of money would be saved, and an awful lot of heartache too.

Renal causes of cystitis are serious. The patient who runs a temperature with the attack must certainly have full urological investigation, because there is always the possibility of future renal damage and failure. When the kidneys don't work the patient doesn't work!

4 Some letters

This idea of printing letters from patients is a great help in cheering them up. They lose the feeling of isolation which is so common in urinary ailments. Urine is a most difficult word to mention to relatives and friends and the whole subject is an embarrassment. To read of other people in the same boat has, I think, been one of the most heartening experiments in our magazine.

A cross-section is here included, together with some medical letters, too, and as I receive approximately 6,000 letters a year you can appreciate the difficulty I have encountered in choosing such a small selection.

Dear U,
At last, I thought, someone really cares! I have suffered from cystitis since childhood; I'm now 38, and have never yet been given any satisfactory answers to its cause.

In the summer I had a nervous breakdown and am now fully recovered, but with yet another bad cystitis attack, I can feel the old depression creeping on, in spite of the drugs I still take for it. I feel I am basically a well-balanced person, but that some physical reason brings on the depression.

Dear U,
I wouldn't risk the experience again for the richest man in the world! I still get cold shivers down my spine when I think about the hell of those ghastly years—dating from the early days of my honeymoon. Never again!

My sympathy goes out to all those women who so suffer, and I would advise them to look for the source of the trouble *very* seriously, as I did, even though the answer is so unpalatable—as in my case.

I don't think there is a more distressing and painful complaint than cystitis, and only those who have suffered from it can fully understand the misery it can cause.

Dear U,
I read with interest your article in the *Sunday Times* of 17-10-71. I suffered from chronic cystitis for over five years and, indeed, it helped to break up my marriage. However, what I cannot accept is that I have to live with this throughout my life. I am at the moment very, very depressed. I had a second IVP last November which was also clear, and a third only two weeks ago. I get very frightened when I have to go for these checks and often feel like suicide.

Dear U,
All the best of luck in your venture. By golly, if only we can find out the cause of this trouble. I've been to two hospitals and just get told: 'You have a germ'. After twelve years I'm really fed up with it.

Dear U,
I have tried your quick method of getting rid of the pain of cystitis and have found it very effective—I can't tell you how grateful I am.

Dear U,
I am 50 and suffered my first attack of this most demoralizing malady shortly after I married in my early twenties. I was talented in many ways but my life has been dogged and diminished as a result of this recurrent trouble. It has, and still

does, hang over my head like the proverbial Sword of Damocles. On this coming Tuesday I have to enter hospital for yet another cystoscopy. Belsen and Dachau could not have been much worse! To say that one's morale drops to point zero is an understatement. I hope that more will be written upon this very painful, depressing and obscure subject, to which it appears little or no research has been devoted.

Dear U,

Please accept £1 as a contribution towards the research programme, instead of requiring the sale of the enclosed tickets. I should only buy them myself, and not even my husband knows I am a member of this club. If I had to explain to people what the club is, and why I need to be a member, the secret that we two have kept for all these years might leak out. Everyone thinks we have a very good marriage, but the truth is that it has been largely sex-less, because of my disability (I can only call it that), and therefore rather empty, many times frustrating, and all rather a waste, especially from my husband's point of view. I would do nothing to give away the fact that he has been so deprived, I should never forgive myself if his men friends ever knew. Our parents never knew, and I have never made close friends in case a possible confidence should be betrayed. We ceased to discuss it long ago ourselves even, so much has our personal relationship suffered. I was anxious for information more than anything else, I know there is no help for my own personal case now.

Dear U,

As was said in your article, the worst aspect of cystitis—apart from the physical pain of the sufferer, is the damaging effect it has on the relationship between two people who love each other. I must be echoing the words of many fellow-sufferers when I say that I feel so hopeless and so low because I see no end to it. This does not mean that I am unaware of the far greater pain and suffering of other people who do not have the good health, happiness and loving home that I am blessed with, but to each person his own pain is the worst and unique. I feel especially sad that it mars my relationship with the person I dearly love and forces me to withdraw more and more, thus making him feel a failure and that my pain is his fault. I am sorry to have written such a long and rather personal letter but I felt I must add yet another voice of support to your fight. How many other women throughout history have suffered this way? And if they have, how strange that it should only be recently that cystitis has even been publicly mentioned. I should like to thank you for trying to do something to awaken the medical world to our desperate plight.

Dear U,

I could hardly believe my ears when I switched on *Woman's Hour*, quite by chance, and heard that splendid lady talking with candour and frankness of the problems of urinary infections related to sexual intercourse.

I too have been struggling with this problem and appreciate all too well the associated difficulties. I should like to applaud this attempt to bring the whole subject out into the open, and feel sure that there will be many who will have been encouraged by the broadcast. Even the feeling of not being the only one similarly afflicted is a great relief!

Dear U,

I am quite sure that the problems in a family home are many where urinary infection is present in one of the parents, and of course, particularly the father as the breadwinner; but that still leaves the other partner with access to breadwinning abilities.

I am unmarried and I have supported myself as best I can

for most of my working life, until I contracted cystitis some five years ago. Since then I have had much time off from my job and my employers have lost profitable working hours. I have now reached such a condition that I am having to consider leaving work altogether. How am I going to live without a regular pay-packet? I have ten years to go before I should retire, so obviously I shan't get a pension. My savings are not enough to last to the end of ten years, let alone to the end of my life, and I find I have a great envy of the married status. I am, to all intents and purposes, disabled, but you wouldn't know it to look at me. I don't need a wheelchair, I am not blind or deaf, and I don't have an illness from which I shall eventually die—nevertheless I am disabled. Could I get a disabled person's pension?

Dear U,
How can I thank you for your leaflet received today, I feel ten years younger already, you so exactly explain the position.

For six years I have suffered. Only yesterday I slunk into the doctor's (and slunk is the word). It is a husband and wife practice. The wife considers my trouble to be 'emotional', and has no time for me; whilst her husband doles out antibiotics (you name it, I've had it) hoping never to see me again.

If only doctors would explain that they are unable to effect a real cure, and explain as you have done the real position, it would be of some comfort. One gets so low and depressed with the pain, that at times I have thought I must have cancer of the bladder, and can go on no longer.

I have been bemoaning my fate that I am only 53 years old, and will I never get better, whilst you are obviously a much younger person, which I think is terrible. Let us hope that something will come of your wonderful venture, and this wonderful thing you are doing.

I make my own barley water, here is the recipe:

A packet of barley flakes, from a health store
2 tablespoons of barley
A little sugar
Covered with about 3 cups of boiling water.
Allow to stand for about 10 minutes, strain off, and drink
whilst hot.

Once again a sincere thank you.

Dear U,
My experience, having been a sufferer from cystitis, may be of
interest to you. Some years ago I got my first attack; some
time elapsed before my next—but then it really hit me so
badly that I was put on Furandantin pills—course three weeks,
one week free, again more pills—this continued and I began to
feel desperate. I do not like pills in any form—I fear too many
would cause side-effects, and my nerves were affected. My
doctor sent me into hospital for an examination and kidney
X-ray. The bladder, I was told, had a slight scar which, when
infected, could be the cause. Kidneys got the all clear. Shortly
after leaving hospital I got another attack—more pills.

Now for the miracle. I have always had a glass of water
before retiring. One night I started drinking and, after
swallowing a couple of mouthfuls, I realized it was overdosed
with chlorine. That night I was awakened with the most
horrible feeling and sensation—and very much pain. It
suddenly struck me—could it be the water I had taken before
bed? There and then I vowed never to drink another drop of
the town's water supply. After that attack I have been free—
over two years now.

I am fortunate in being able to get beautiful spring water
coming down from a mountain near my home. I still use town
supply for cooking—the chlorine can be boiled out; but when

they add fluoride I will have to stop, because it is deadly for
kidney and bladder complaints.

My case surely proves the danger to older people of adding
medicaments to the water supply—by the way I am now 65
years old.

Hoping that perhaps you or your fellow-sufferers may get
some relief by avoiding the town's water supply.

Dear U,
I listened at 12 noon today to the talk on cystitis, though I do
not know why they called it unmentionable—I mention it all
the time! I thought you might be interested in my own
experiences.

The surgeons finally diagnosed 'Interstitial Cystitis', and I
had my bladder stretched, under anaesthetic, ten times
altogether, since 1967. Then in 1969 they decided to cut the
top off the bladder, since that was where the ulcers were. This
would, they said, make it smaller, but it might stretch again,
and anyway I would have no pain. So they cut my tum from
navel to pelvis and cut off the top, but after six months I was
worse than before. The small bladder hadn't stretched, the
ulcers had returned, and quite truthfully, I could not walk to
the end of the road.

Then they said I could have the thing removed and wear an
external bag, or they were willing to try, if my family
approved, a new technique of removing all but the base of the
bladder and using part of my intestine as a bladder; but they
guaranteed nothing, and said they couldn't work miracles. I
said, if it fails, and all the operation is for nothing again, why
don't you give me the bag straight away, but they said, 'Oh
this way is much better, if it works.' Well, I didn't really see
why my family had to approve, as I am 61, and anyway I
hoped, really hoped that I would die under the anaesthetic, so
I had it done. It took ages, I was out of the world from 1.30 to

7.30 and the sisters and interested medicos watched from the gallery (but they said they couldn't see much, the heads kept getting in the way!)

Well, it worked. I can now usually last for two hours. I do still get up in the night, sometimes only twice, but sometimes quite often, but I can go shopping and return without looking for a loo.

The water is very cloudy, and always will be, because it has passed through the intestines, but they are pleased with me and I look extremely healthy. But I still get a pain, a squeezing pain, about every half-hour. I haven't got to go to see the surgeon for four months.

Dear U,

I have read of your Club in the *Sunday Times* and should be interested in any information or help you give to sufferers. I feel doubly qualified since I myself first had cystitis some ten months ago, and have had about a dozen similar attacks since. Also, more important to me at the moment is my daughter's case. At $2\frac{1}{2}$ years she has this September been *very* ill and was admitted to hospital with an undiagnosed complaint, which turned out to be urinary infection. She has had various tests and investigations and, although well in herself, is still under care of the out-patients at hospital, and will have to be on antibiotics for long term. I was told she must be kept on the medicine indefinitely or else the infection will recur and could spread to the kidneys. It is most worrying for me that she should, at this age, have to be on medicine, and also that they have told me she should just grow out of it, which seems rather vague.

Dear U,

To put it mildly, male ignorance about sexual hygiene is abysmal. To quote from a recent survey: 'In men penile hygiene was appalling and lack of knowledge was not confined to school children. Among the latter only 8 out of 10 uncircumcised boys even knew about the necessity of washing behind the prepuce. Basically the argument revolves round the findings that over 80% of school leavers are ignorant of even the basis of penile hygiene.' To quote from another: 'The ignorance of these young men is remarkable; many of them expressed surprise at the condition revealed when they retracted their foreskins.'

It is true to say that more constructive thought should be given as much to the prevention as to the treatment of urogenital infection. Moralizing gets us nowhere, particularly when it is evident that previously accepted codes of conduct are substantially rejected. Personal hygiene is basic prophylaxis, but it is a subject that more than most is governed by taboos and inhibitions. A lead should be given by the Ministries of Health and Education.

Dear U,

I would like to make two points:

1 Scandinavian doctors claim that many women are sensitive to most ordinary soaps, that such soap can help bring the condition about, and may keep it alive for years. Thus they recommend that you stop using soap in the area altogether.

2 It is known by quite a few (old-fashioned) doctors in Britain that the application of witchhazel will often remove pain. They still, of course give their patients antibiotics, but my own experience with witchhazel is remarkable. After two years of agony, the pain disappeared within half-a-second, literally. At first it may be necessary to repeat the application each time one has been to the toilet. It should be pressed into the urethra with a small piece of cotton wool. Chronic sufferers might be advised to take a small bottle of witchhazel with them everywhere, for perhaps a few months.

Dear U,
I suffer from a bladder complaint which is now proving a
great handicap to my husband and myself. Between 1950 and
1960 I had three 'plastic repair' operations, with months of
subsequent bladder misery, and now cannot seem to travel any
distance more than about 20 miles by car or train without
symptoms occurring similar to those of cystitis. These
symptoms do not clear when travelling stops but, once
triggered off, can take weeks to clear. I do suffer from true
cystitis too, but cannot tell the difference in the symptoms. All
holidays taken in this country during the last five years have
been a misery, thinking I had cystitis, and swallowing masses
of antibiotics, before we discovered that it has been caused by
the vibration of travelling.
    I have to have tranquillizers and anti-depressants to help
clear it up, but they do not prevent it; it still occurred during a
course of anti-depressants on only a 30-minute trip.
    I have used a Dunlopillo cushion with a hole in the middle
for years, which helps but does not by any means prevent the
effects of vibration, and the distance which I can travel seems
to get less each year.
    My doctor tells me that he has never known of anyone else
affected in the same way, and I am very interested to know if
there are any other readers who do.

Dear U,
In addition to my own troubles, my daughter, now eight, had
her first bout when she was three. They were often quite
serious, leading to much pain and high fevers. She had gone
into Children's Hospital Medical Centre in Boston on two
occasions for cystoscopy, fluoroscopy, etc. The only
conclusion has been that she suffers from reflux, but that
corrective surgery is not called for. Consequently she has been
on Gantrisin therapy off and on for four years; the last session

with Gantrisin went on for eight months. I can't believe this is good for a child although the doctor reassures me that there are no side-effects. I remain dubious and would seek other remedies. But, of course, I'm no 'expert' and we do tend to defer to them.

Your journal is a splendid idea because it involves education and self-help. I believe it would improve the quality of medical care enormously if we became intelligent patients. I'm convinced this helps keep doctors on their toes!

I might add that another great problem associated with frequent illness and drug therapy in the States is the high costs associated with them. We have no national health care and exorbitant fees are charged by doctors and for medication. With a family of four children we spend over $1000 yearly—and this involves no *major* accidents, injuries, illnesses. It's outrageous, really.

Dear U,
You have my everlasting gratitude for the Bicarb tip. I take ½ teaspoon daily and have been free from the dreadful scourge for 17 weeks. Why can't doctors, before entering on the everlasting tablets business, suggest this?

Dear U,
Keep up the good work. Enclosed please find cheque for £3—my subscription plus a little extra. Have enjoyed my most cystitis-free year for nearly sixteen years—many thanks.

Dear U,
I have been shown Anne Allen's piece from the *Sunday Mirror* concerning the U and I Club. In the course of this article, there is a reference to men 'with bothersome prostatitis'.

Unfortunately, I am plagued by just such a condition. After long bouts of great discomfort which necessitated absence from my work, my doctor was persuaded to arrange hospital tests. Investigation took the form of X-rays, cystoscopy and sigmoidoscopy and the result was (I felt) rather vague diagnosis of colitis, prostatitis and signs of urethritis.

I am completely in the dark as to the cause of my trouble and cannot pin-point any likely time it could have begun. My doctor and also the hospital specialists have been equally vague and it has slowly dawned on me that this is because they don't know. Worry made me attend the VD clinic where they again found prostatitis, but cleared me of any condition which came in their sphere.

I am looking forward to my first real holiday in over two years—I hope to go to Spain in two weeks time—but have again been troubled by the nagging aches in the loins, the pain in the lower back, etc. My doctor, whom I consulted today, has at last been frank with me. I told him I was becoming philosophic about my condition and thought I could now cope with it, but hope it would not get any worse. Was it possible that it could get better? His answer was 'No'. Not at present. He explained that because this condition was becoming increasingly common, a great deal of research was now being done. It was important to 'maintain my condition'. He gave a parallel—insulin for diabetics. The drug I am at present provided with is Urolocosil, which I am to take when I feel the attack coming on. I cannot truthfully say I find it of value. I also have a supply of Sulphadimidine which I rely on to stay the rather severe diarrhoea which seems to come on with the inflammation. Usually I am forced to retire to bed, where I seem to sleep night and day until the system settles itself. I have noticed that getting physically chilled seems to be one way the attacks are triggered. I am wondering whether your organization can offer any more practical advice on heading off attacks (especially in view of my approaching holiday!)

Dear U,

I have had several urine tests, and my doctor assures me that no infection is present and that there is nothing further he can do. This leaves me 'high and dry' (no play on words intended!). I am completely unable to have any social life–I would dearly love to go to the pictures or the theatre, but past trips have caused me so much misery that I no longer try. Even in a place where a toilet is easily accessible, e.g. someone's house, I suffer agony rather than keep asking to visit the 'loo'. No one would object to my disappearing once in an evening, but three or four times is ridiculous. At work I am in an office where a trip to the 'Ladies' takes me past about twenty men's desks–and you can imagine the remarks, which vary from 'She's been on the beer again' to, on a very cold day, 'I wish your plumbing would freeze'. I laugh, I have to; but inside I'm really in tears–this really is ruining my whole life and stopping me from making friends–how can you explain to a stranger (especially a man) that you have to make a half-hourly exit (more frequent sometimes)?

Dear U,

I thought you might be interested to know that I have had a 'trouble-free' *six months*, after many attacks in quick succession. My doctor suggested that I took one 100gm tablet of Furadantin directly after intercourse. I also drink about ½ pint of water and then urinate. So far so good!

Every success to the U and I.

Dear U,

I have just finished reading the article about cystitis in *Woman* magazine.

As I am at the moment suffering my sixth attack, you will understand I found that article very interesting. I have either visited my doctor, or rung, on each occasion but have never as yet been examined; each time he prescribed a course of tablets and told me to take all of them, but apart from that I have had no advice at all, nor would he visit on occasions when I have been too ill to go to surgery. My husband has been told to go and collect my prescription.

After reading the article in *Woman* I realize just how much could have been done for me, especially as this last attack has been bothering me for almost a week and shows no sign of clearing. I am now about to get ready to visit my doctor and demand an examination and better treatment.

Dear Madam,

Thank you very much for your full and interesting letter and your suggestions with regard to the development of some sort of collective action to combat this problem of urinary infection in women. I have taken the liberty of discussing your letter with my colleagues. They feel, as I do myself, that probably the first step would be to meet you and discuss some of the problems of this condition as they appear to us from the medical side and then try to work out how we could best cooperate for the benefit of the many women afflicted by this disease.

I would suggest that the best thing you could do would be to come to St — Hospital on a Friday afternoon at about 4 o'clock to meet the Consultants concerned during their normal weekly Urinary Infection Conference. Let me know when this would be convenient to you and we will all arrange to be there and discuss the matter.

I would be very keen myself on some sort of news sheet as the more propaganda we can get disseminated about this

distressing condition and its management the better, and I have a few ideas myself. I think we could best discuss them together rather than trying to communicate rather long-windedly through the post.
Consultant Urologist

Dear Madam,
I was very interested to read in a recent issue of the *Sunday Times* the article concerning cystitis and your charity organization, the U and I Club. I am a clinical microbiologist and for many years I have taken a particular interest in urinary tract infections.

I agree with many of your statements and views concerning cystitis but I would like to suggest a few points which your charity organization may consider.

1 Urinary tract infections may be symptomatic or asymptomatic. Both are equally important in the aetiological aspects of the infection although symptomatic infection is only important to the woman. Similarly most general practitioners are unconcerned about asymptomatic infections.

2 There is no one form of urinary tract infection and consequently no single form of treatment will be effective in all women with cystitis.

3 Although many facts about urinary tract infection have been known for over a century, the basic reason why some women are prone to this condition is not known. In some circles of clinicians the interest shown in urinary tract infections is waning and it would be a pity if the basic causes for cystitis were not discovered.

With regard to your point about embarrassment discussing urinary troubles, I think this is primarily concerned with the apparent interest of the doctor. I find no problems discussing aspects of the patient's sexual activity or urinary symptoms probably because I am sympathetic and convinced of the importance of appropriate and correct treatment.

In conclusion I think it is vitally important that cystitis is discussed from a medical and scientific background. It is essential that the correct treatment and follow-up is instigated and that bacteriological tests are carried out where possible in all cases of cystitis.
Consultant Microbiologist

Dear Madam,
Two of your magazines have been handed to me to read by a patient, and I have read them with considerable interest.

I am a General Surgeon, but 80% of my work is Urology and I am particularly interested in this problem. I have one or two ideas that I may wish to contribute to your magazine one day.

First of all, however, I would like to join the U and I Club and I would like copies of all the magazines published so far. I enclose a cheque for £3, which I hope will cover the membership fee and the cost of sending the magazines. If there is a balance left over, please keep it for your trouble.
General Surgeon

Dear Madam,
I think that the work you are doing is of the greatest importance and I hope that this will be the start of a fruitful collaboration. I feel sure that any study of urinary infection must be outward-looking and go to the community. This is the approach that we have now been making for a number of years. I am very much looking forward to meeting you.
Professor of Pathology

Dear Madam,
I read with interest your letter in the *Lancet* of 29 January and would like to congratulate you on your enterprise in giving

publicity to this very common problem from which you
and, I have no doubt, hundreds of thousands of women suffer.

As you are probably aware a considerable amount of
research into the problem is going on but it is also true to say
that we are not much further on in coming to any conclusion.
It may encourage you to know that I certainly make it my
business to teach all students that come through our
department what is known about this disease and to ensure
that all of them are in possession of the valuable 'penny
spending tip' which does so much to make life more bearable
for a lot of women.
Consultant in Venereology

Dear Madam,
I am sure there is a huge group of people who could benefit
from joining (judging from your bi-monthly magazine) and
if I come across a few of them I will try to get them to belong.

I am really very impressed with your enterprise and
enormous efforts and drive.

I am the consultant Mr — approached you about. (I am a
child psychiatrist but also very interested in the problems of
the mentally handicapped too.) I am also a recurrent cystitis
sufferer as well as being a doctor, and assiduously study the
BMJ, etc, for new ideas. To be honest, apart from antibiotics
and antiseptics, I have read more useful advice and information
on the subject of this wretched complaint from your 'U and I'
than I have done over the years in medical journals!! Really,
this is rather disgraceful but it does highlight the benefit
of your own endeavours.
Psychiatrist

Dear Madam,
I note in the *Sunday Times* of 24 October that your
organization has been set up for sufferers from cystitis.

As a Physician with a special interest in renal disease I was interested to hear of your organization and would appreciate you sending me details of your aims and objectives and also copies of any information you may send to interested people or members.

It is obviously important that I should be aware of these facts as a significant part of my practice is concerned with the care and treatment of this condition.
Consultant Physician

Dear Madam,
Some time ago I saw with interest your article in the London *Times*. Today, I was reading your letter in the January 29th *Lancet* and I wish to establish contact with you.

I am an Infectious Disease Microbiologist interested in urinary infection for the past 6 years. My work to date has been primarily in exploring mechanisms of recurrence in females with recurrent disease. Your thoughts on the importance of hormonal balance in urinary infection are interesting. Obviously, they need to be explored. My major investigation at present is trying to document perineal flora in women with recurrent infections. This does indeed appear to be different than women who do not get recurrences, that is, young married women with recurrences tend to have large numbers of gram negative organisms on their perineum and often Enterococci, whereas normal women, not prone to urinary infection, rarely have these potential urinary pathogens on their perineum and their vagina. Perhaps, the bacterial ecology of the perineum may be determined by hormonal influences on the vagina and perineum.

I am specifically writing to ask if you have any clubs on this side of the Atlantic. I have approximately 75 women in my study with recurring infection and I am sure they would benefit by a club similar to that you have founded. Could I refer several of my patients to your club officials in order that they might acquire more information on the organization and objective of your club? I do think your advice and encouragement to this population of unfortunate women is indeed of value.

Clinical Microbiologist

Dear Madam,

I was glad to hear that you had set up the U and I Club. I regard cystitis and other forms of urinary tract inflammation as a very important and very neglected cause of illness among the adult female population.

In 1963–4 we made a survey of the incidence of clinically recognizable urinary tract inflammation in this practice and found that 6·2 per cent of the total practice population was affected at some time during that twelve months.

Female: Male proportion 4·5:1.

Last year I made a personal survey among my own patients and found that 10 per cent of all my 'items of service'—consultations and visits—were concerned with this condition. I was delighted to note your paragraph in *GP* (Feb 2nd) concerning the social, family and psychological effects of this illness and was able to make good use of it in a tutorial I gave to junior doctors in Norwich this week. Your findings are compatible with my own in this field though I must confess to having overlooked the effect of cystitis on female employment. I enclose £1 as a contribution to the expenses of your organization.

General Practitioner

5 The sexual organs

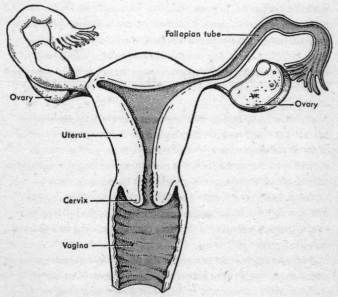

Ovaries, uterus, vagina

It is a constant source of amazement to me that this relatively small set of organs can be removed and yet the patient still lives!

Take away the heart, lungs, kidneys or liver and you die. Yet the ovaries and uterus are important enough to be the mainstay of the human race and are probably a woman's main cause of concern for her bodily health.

It is very important that these organs are constantly healthy. Our doctors seem to pay great attention, and rightly so, in matters of childbirth, abortion and hysterectomy, but much more could be done for the smaller ailments which affect the sexual organs. Just like others they are prone to infections, inflammation, deformities and general weaknesses.

How many women for instance wander around with bad periods, backache, nervous tension, anaemia? Not a lot of attention is paid to them. Mostly they are told to forget it; 'it will get better after you are married; it will get better after your children are born; it will get better when you have finished the menopause; what can you expect at your age; buy yourself some Iron Jelloids,' and finally, 'you're imagining it!'

Anaemia is woman's ever-present enemy. The amount of blood that some women lose each month is very close to the amount necessary for a wounded soldier to receive almost instant blood transfusion! Yet the woman goes on month after month thinking it is nearly normal (a) because one never actually sees the amount other friends lose and (b) because blood tests are not a routine occurrence. I should like to see every woman attend a clinic three times a year for blood tests whether pregnant or not.

Perhaps again I can enlighten the reader from some personal experience. In my time I too have experienced these lengthy, heavy periods. Now, my private GP would first send me for a free and fast blood test at the Middlesex Hospital and then, without waiting, would give an intravenous iron injection of some 5cc once or even twice a week until he was sure that I was back up again in the 80s and 90s. An important point to remember here is that some people have allergic reactions to intravenous iron injections and that a small 'test' dose is necessary in order to allay any fear that this might be the case.

One winter he was away in South Africa and my NHS doctor was the only person to whom I could go. I was terribly ill that winter with five virus lung infections, ten colds, six stomach bugs, cystitis and heavy periods. I looked terrible, felt awful and finally the GP said that he would give me an iron injection with extra vitamin content. Well, when it arrived I could hardly see the fluid in the container. No mention was made of a blood test, and only on the return of my private GP did I receive the necessary treatment. You just take a look at the number of white-faced, lethargic women around, particularly in large towns, and you'll see just why iron injections should be given more readily.

What causes a woman to lose enough blood to become anaemic? Well funnily enough it may be anaemia!

All muscles are fed by blood and its ingredients. If they are incorrectly fed the muscles will not have sufficient strength to support each organ. Thus it happens that the organs can also become tired, and when the blood lining of the uterus breaks away once a month to begin menstruation a lot more comes away than should do because of tired muscle reaction.

Secondly the uterus also reacts upon the oestrogen/ progestogen messages from the pituitary gland via the ovaries. If these messages are too profuse then the uterus receives instructions to release more and more blood! In other words the messengers are imbalanced!

My private GP has always stated that if more care was given to hormone imbalance and iron, then hysterectomies would be less necessary. Even nowadays, with the advent of the contraceptive pill which usually alleviates the monthly blood loss, there are still specialists who feel that the answer to heavy periods is to remove the uterus. Removal of both uterus and ovaries is another kind of hysterectomy used when all previous treatment has apparently failed, but again, the resulting cessation of hormone supply can prove difficult. A quotation by Ovid is very apt in this sense,

Too late is the medicine prepared
When the disease has gained strength by long delays.

When the blood iron-count is high, resistance to all sorts of infections is also high, including urinary infection. Being tired means that you cannot cope so well with cystitis either mentally or physically. They are extremely wearing symptoms to cope with apart from whatever cause is lurking in the background, and it pays dividends to ensure that you are living a regular and healthy life.

Backache, tension, irritability and depression can also be caused by anaemia, but again it is of the highest importance for the doctor to make some attempt to check up the progestogen/oestrogen hormone balance. Depression in cystitis really comes under the chapter headed 'Stress', but depression is definitely associated with anaemia and hormone imbalance—tranquillizers are not the only answer and no patient should blindly accept such drugs as a treatment.

American researchers have produced a hormone test, but because it is so new it is a very expensive procedure. In England our scientists are at much the same sort of stage, but work still continues to find a cheap, fast and accurate way of assessing a woman's hormone balance. At the moment the assessment depends entirely on the skills and experience of each examining gynaecologist. One might spot something that another may not; it's rather unsettling really.

The vagina and cervix are the most easily accessible organs to examine and generally their mucus contents speak quite loudly for their state of health to the competent eye. Certain invading organisms like thrush or trichomonas can be detected from swabs cultured and then viewed under a microscope, so the infections can be accounted for, but the hormonal effect upon the vagina is changeable and more difficult to spot accurately with the naked eye. As we know, there are no swabs or tests available. In the main the women with predominant oestrogen (female) outputs have softer, pliable and more rounded contours to their vaginal tissue, whilst the lack of oestrogen produces roughly the opposite effect. But the variations are individual and only properly discernible by special experience.

The state of the vagina is also going to affect the woman's sexual desire. It is a cruel, outdated, ignorant man nowadays who accuses his wife of frigidity. She simply cannot help herself if her vagina is unresponsive. It may well mean that the chronic vaginal discharge is so bad that nerve-endings fail to cooperate one with another and so the signal impulse is thwarted, the sexual secretions just cannot push a way through the other contents.

The sexual organs unfortunately lie so close to the bladder and urethra that what affects one affects the other. A full bladder can inhibit easy intercourse—a prolapsed uterus can inhibit easy bladder function.

Likewise, it has been proved in research that the same hormonal changes in menopausal women can also cause thickening of the urethral tissues. These changes take place all over the body and there is no reason why the urethra should be left out! The condition is known as distal urethral stenosis and is simply hardening or cornification of the urethral tissue. The vagina secretes very little mucus leaving it susceptible to cracking and infection. One of the most outrageous letters I ever received was from a menopausal woman whose GP had stated that hormone treatment was no use until the age of 75 years because until that time the treatment would need to be continuous. It is unbelievable that a registered GP with such an outlook should be practising in the British Isles. One cannot lay down hard and fast rules because each woman is so distinct in her make-up. Some need a tiny course, others, like me, need to watch and treat the hormone balance continually.

Years ago we were all told that women grew hairy faces and chests if hormones were administered. This is old wives' mushy rubbish, but it has unfortunately lingered on because no one has bothered to re-educate us. You will not grow a beard and if you are treated correctly and under constant good medical supervision you will feel much, much better, not so depressed, generally healthier, even sexually healthier with better periods.

I believe that from the age of thirteen years or so a woman's hormone balance needs observing and is of the utmost importance in keeping her healthy. It is time this country realized that its excessive tranquillizer bill and its high female suicide rate is not only unnecessary but indicative of some uninformed doctoring.

6 The renal organs

We are often made aware of how our sexual organs work but for the urinary patient it is also necessary to have a rudimentary knowledge of how the renal organs work.

We must also know what the blood contains because it is the blood and its contents which flow into the kidneys. Blood is the carrier of our life. Without it we die. Roughly, we all have eight pints of it flowing through every artery, vein, muscle and organ in our body. Its duties are manifold: to convey proteins, water, heat, red and white corpuscles, hormones of all sorts, carbon dioxide, oxygen, acids, poisons, iron and a multitude of broken-down foods, minerals, bacteria and organisms to and from the major organs, muscles, glands and the brain. It's the body's railway network!

The kidneys have the job of sorting out what is needed and what can be discarded, and the female's kidneys are smaller than those of the male.

Blood flows into each kidney through the renal artery to all the various parts of the kidneys via many tiny arterioles which wrap themselves around thousands of minute tubules. Here in the tubules the sifting and sorting out of the blood's ingredients is done. If the tubules discover too much water, salt, urea, uric acid or other substances they absorb them from the bloodstream and then eject them through the ureter in the liquid form of urine. The corrected blood is then transferred into venules, passed out of the kidney via the renal vein and back again to the main bloodstream.

Meanwhile urine filters out through the two long, fine

pipes called ureters and drops down through a valve in each of them into the bladder. As the urine descends, this valve, when working properly, opens on the stimulus of the urine itself. When all that particular batch of urine has passed through, the valve closes for a while until the next batch arrives. If it doesn't close properly, or closes too quickly, stale urine can be squirted back up towards the kidneys. The impurities and organisms remain in it for a while and over a period of time infection can set in.

However, let us assume that all is in order. The bladder, into which the urine passes and where it is stored for a while, is a hollow muscular sac capable of holding about half a pint of urine, perhaps a little more. As the urine level rises the bladder expands and stimulates the sensory nerve fibres within the bladder wall. When capacity level is reached the stimulus reminds the brain that it is time to empty the bladder.

If it happens to be inconvenient to empty the bladder at the time this signal is sent, then it is possible consciously to tell the bladder not to empty itself, but the higher the urine pressure rises, stretching the bladder further, the more impossible it is to 'hold it', and the more harm may result.

Once the decision is made to 'release' and pass the water, two things happen.

The valve leading into the exit passage or urethra is called the sphincter and as we relax to allow the urine to flow, so this sphincter valve is also relaxed, and allows the urine to pass through into the urethra. If this sphincter does not work correctly the urine trickles through constantly and the patient is known as incontinent. The valve may only be partly deficient so that urine escapes when the patient sneezes, coughs or laughs.

At the same time as the healthy sphincter opens, the bladder's muscular wall contracts and pushes the urine out.

When it has all been passsed, the sphincter closes up and the storage process begins all over again. In a normal person this happens four or five times a day and not at all during the night. Obviously it depends on how much and what you have been drinking.

What about the positioning of these organs? Well, in the female, as our diagram shows below, the urethra runs almost parallel to the vagina and, as we already know, the vaginal and urethral orifices are extremely close to one another, even *affecting* and *infecting* one another.

In the male the same tubular exit pipe is used for urine and semen, although not at the same time providing all the various valves are working properly! (diagram page 68)

Obviously the nervous system plays an important part in the normality of micturition (the act of passing urine). The bladder wall nerve fibres, as previously discussed, ensure that the bladder muscles push out all the stored urine. This network of nerve fibres receives instructions from other sets of nerves which in turn receive orders from the lumbosacral spinal cord. So long as this is intact and able to receive the initial brain message then micturition can still take place on

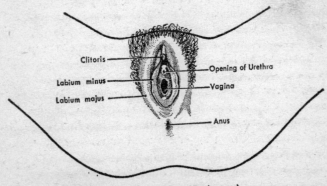

Vagina and urethra and their orifices (Perineum)

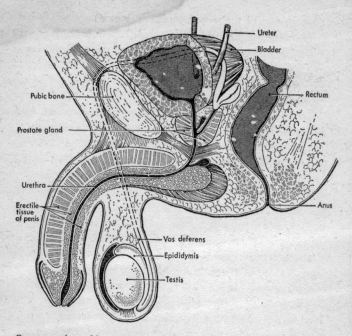

Ureter
Bladder
Pubic bone
Rectum
Prostate gland
Urethra
Anus
Erectile tissue of penis
Vas deferens
Epididymis
Testis

Cross-section of internal penis relating to prostate and testicles

the reflex. If damage or obstruction of messages takes place en route between the brain and the bladder then the bladder cannot begin to empty itself unless helped further. Sometimes this can be done by applying hot or cold sponged water to excite and stimulate the bladder nerve fibres, or by catheterization. Someone with an injured lower spinal cord can be advised about either of these methods by a neurologist and urologist once an estimate has been made of the extent of the damage.

A diabetic's main problem is that the nervous system responds adversely to the high amount of glucose which is symptomatic to the ailment. In regard to the bladder

mechanism it is again the nerve fibres which are damaged.
The result is rather contradictory with either incontinence or
water retention. The sphincter valve refuses to work because
there are no nerve impulses to tell it to! So it either stays
permanently shut or permanently open, responding generally
to the insertion of a catheter.

Renal failure, unlike failure of the sexual organs, can result
in death. It is virtually impossible to tell early enough that a
patient's kidneys are on the road to 'extremis' because the
symptoms are so vague. Anaemia, tiredness, breathlessness,
nausea, occasional blood loss and passing of extra large
amounts of water are symptomatic. Only when the symptoms
are really acute can the process of failure be detected by the
screening processes. Once the problem is discovered, the
patient can nowadays be kept alive on a kidney machine. Renal
dialysis, as it is called, is the process of artificially cleansing
the blood by passing it through a machine for 24 hours.
This is generally done twice a week with the patient either
hospitalized in a special unit or, with a lot of financial assistance,
in a specially converted room at home. Occasionally a
patient may be lucky enough to have a kidney transplant if
both kidneys have failed to work. A donor is found, either
dead or alive, to give a kidney for transplantation to the
affected patient. It must be pointed out, however, that a
great many people live comfortably on one good kidney with
only a slight easing-up of life's pace.

Thus it is of paramount importance that at least we stop
ascending infections from adding to the kidneys' problems.
Constant pyelitis, as previously pointed out, can be dangerous
and must be controlled. All simple urinary infections, if not
prevented, managed and controlled, may ascend and involve
the kidneys. Cystitis, even in its simplest form, must **never**
be ignored.

7 Stress

How often do we hear this word in the twentieth century! Cars, trains, noise, small living quarters, aeroplanes, jobs, double lives—anything and everything. There is so much to do, to see, to hear. Certain conformities with society still arise and we have to 'keep up with it'. Great happiness, great sorrow, annoyances, quarrels, home-hunting, moving, illness—you name it—it's there in everybody's life.

Well what exactly is stress? How does it affect our physical bodies?

Stress can be defined perhaps as that situation where excesses in or extremes of emotional feeling are aroused.

The immediate effect of it is to excite any given part of the receptive brain into taking positive action. The brain then sends out nerve impulses or hormone messengers to the appropriate organ or muscle telling it to get on with the job it was designed to do, i.e. lift an arm to strike someone or something, become verbally excited, become sexually excited, cry, laugh, the items are endless.

Sometimes, in fact quite often, the stress builds up because the pressure is working over a period of time, i.e. build-up to the wedding day and honeymoon, illness leading to death, family arguments, build-up to divorce, maybe just office worries and decision-making (and, most definitely, book-writing!)

The ability to cope with it depends on how much stability your character and personality has, how easily you can adapt to a situation—but even then one's balance is initially, albeit temporarily, overthrown according to the ferocity of the situation.

Immediate reactions can be fear, nausea, vomiting, tears, urination, even temporary unconsciousness. Distant reactions can be withdrawal from reality, bad periods in women, high blood-pressure, ulcers, bladder problems, tenseness, depression, cystitis, suicide, to name but a few.

In other words a mental situation can lead to a physical reaction.

I once had a letter published in the *Lancet* about stress in relation to cystitis and the urethral syndrome. Now the urethral syndrome is the name given by the medical profession to a group of quite unaccountable urinary symptoms that appear to have no cause. It mystifies and puzzles many a young or ageing medical brain, and various methods of treating it have been attempted with many a failure. All tests and examinations seem to prove negative and the patient is often told: 'You're imagining it, go away and tell yourself it doesn't exist.' The patient, fearing for sanity, gets more and more alarmed and worried as further attacks occur. The stress weighs heavily and not just on the patient – I know of a young woman whose sufferings triggered off her father's first coronary; her husband began to lose concentration at work and inevitably their marriage and family suffered.

This, unfortunately, is fairly common. Whatever the cause, if it is not rooted out quickly, the recurrence of symptomatic cystitis will begin a stress build-up.

However, I have strayed a little from my *Lancet* letter. I received fifteen letters from Consultants and GPs, some from abroad, in interested comment and agreement. Basically my points were these:

stress causes functional changes in the ovaries – stress such as on honeymoon, trauma on assumption of regular intercourse, childbirth, occasionally in menopause and after hysterectomy and, of course, all other situations in life. Ovarian changes affect the hormonal content of the vagina resulting in greater or fewer secretions, e.g. honeymoon sexual excitement and vaginal stimulation. If these secretions are either profuse or minimal the way is open for an unhealthy vagina to accommodate bacteria. The urethra also undergoes these hormonal changes as do other organs in the body; e.g. the heart responds adversely to the kind of hormonal activity which produces higher sugar, fat and carbohydrate levels in the bloodstream. These products are deposited over the years, under stress situations, in and around the heart tissues which eventually become thickened and cease to work correctly.

Much the same thing happens to the vagina—it gets clogged up and cannot work. Urologists seldom examine the vagina—it's not their realm; neither do gynaecologists care much about the urethra. It's about time they did. What a lot of time, money and energy we could save!

So if we take a stress as possibly causing cystitis and this unsolved recurrent cystitis causes stress, then we logically assume that cystitis can cause cystitis, although not initially.

But woe betide the doctor who accepts this as read and does nothing constructive to break up the sequence.

8 Children

I can't write an awful lot about cystitis in children because I don't know very much about it. Certain things I do know though. Cystitis in children has a smaller area of investigation to cover. For instance there is nothing sexual in any way involved; therefore one can concentrate on searching the renal organs for the cause. Once all relevant X-rays have been taken, the urologist either finds some sort of congenital deformity, omission, reflux, or nothing. If one of the three former problems exists then treatment can usually be successfully commenced.

If the urologist finds nothing and urine specimen cultures still show bacteria, then it can be assumed that an ascending infection may be the culprit. In other words hygiene is lax or the child has some sort of allergy or is in contact with an irritant such as Hexachlorophene, which is to be found in a great many bathroom products like soap, shampoo and powder—also deodorants. Check the ingredients mentioned on the packet, tin or aerosol and don't touch any that contain Hexachlorophene.

My small daughter had two mystery bouts of urinary trouble—she cried on micturition, withheld it, and was very sore and inflamed. There were no bacteria in her urine but the bouts all recurred whilst we had in use a bottle of medicated shampoo. The minute it dawned on me, I looked at the bottle and, sure enough, there was Hexachlorophene written. Sometimes the manufacturers turn the letters around and you might see for instance Chlorohexaphene–don't touch it!

Something else to check if recurrent attacks seem constant is your washing powder. As the pants and knickers retaining detergent rub against a child's very tender perineum, allergies can start. It pays to rinse all underwear until the water is perfectly clear, and bleach should be avoided.

Never put antiseptics in the bath, check the soap used and keep bath toys clean. Just don't put anything except clear, clean water in the bath.

Change the underwear every day and if in trouble with cystitis, wash your child's bottom twice a day and *always* after its bowels have moved. Hygiene is vital. Teach it to wipe its bottom from front to back with a soft toilet tissue.

The most common form of childhood bladder problem is bedwetting or enuresis. The social consequences of enuresis may be a breakdown in the interpersonal relationships with a family, resulting in a child becoming a social outcast. The frustrations caused by the continuation of the condition in the child bring despair to the parents. Worry and anxiety particularly affect the mother, who suffers emotional disturbance caused by feelings of inadequacy and the embarrassing problem of the smell involved, as well as the physical strain of extra washing and ironing.

Considerable confusion exists over the definition of enuresis. In this context it is defined as involuntary urination occurring during sleep in children over the age of three years. Enuresis may be divided into primary and secondary types. Primary enuresis is defined as the failure of these children ever to have achieved control of micturition, and secondary enuresis as the onset of enuresis after a period of nocturnal continence of at least one year after the age of three years, this being the age by which most children have acquired continence.

As a generalization it may be said that the incidence of enuresis is 15 per cent at five years old, 5 per cent at ten years old, and 1 per cent at fifteen years old.

These figures reveal the immensity of the problem itself, irrespective of the emotional factors which may result from the primary condition. The child suffers shame and frustration associated with the fear of humiliation should other children discover the secret. Holidays, school journeys and camps are usually denied the children because of the enuresis and much self-limitation may result. A strained relationship between parent and child is a further difficulty which may occur even in a well-adjusted family. Frequently advice is given that 'he will grow out of it', but this is wrong, as thorough follow-ups have produced evidence showing enuresis may not be self-limiting. It is therefore advisable to begin treatment at an early age, and four years of age is suggested as reasonable.

A large number of physical conditions have been reported in the literature as being associated with enuresis, namely meatal stenosis, small bladders, congenital hypertrophy of the bladder neck. It can also be associated with chronic inflammatory change high up in the urethra and neck of the bladder. Despite treatment for these various conditions, however, some doctors consider that the correction of physical defects usually has no effect on established enuresis; and furthermore, the majority of children with enuresis have no such defects.

Considerable evidence has been amassed noting the frequent occurrence of enuresis in other members of an enuretic's family, but an accurate determination is difficult, as tracing and interviewing relatives is often impossible and their memories are by no means reliable.

Deep sleep is frequently cited as a cause of enuresis. The explanation is attractive, for it seems logical that if a child sleeps deeply it will be unable to perceive rising bladder pressure and enuresis will occur; but this reasoning does not explain why other deep-sleeping children have complete nocturnal continence.

Lack of toilet-training during early childhood is often considered a cause for enuresis, whilst, conversely, early or strict training is also implicated.

The majority of enuretic children, when presented for treatment, are not emotionally disturbed. If emotional disturbance exists it need not be relevant to enuresis, and is more likely to be a secondary feature than a prime contributory cause. The stoicism and fortitude of enuretic children commands admiration and it is remarkable that they suffer the misery of a wet bed for long periods and emerge mentally unscathed.

Treatment must be enthusiastic, rejecting despondency. Methods tried include restriction of fluids, 'potting' throughout the night, use of drugs to calm or suppress nervous reactions, but by far the most successful is conditioning treatment.

The enuretic responds to the stimulus of a full bladder by urination. Treatment consists of associating the same stimulus with a wakening stimulus—namely, the operation of an electric bell or buzzer when urination starts. The response of urination is inhibited by wakening and this inhibition of micturition, by a conditioning process, ultimately occurs spontaneously without the necessity of wakening or the operation of the bell or buzzer.

The average duration of treatment is $2-2\frac{1}{2}$ months and the cases of relapse are given a second course of treatment. Although many children have been successfully treated, more research is needed to solve unanswered problems.

9 Medical investigations

As we know there are two major lines of investigation into the cause of cystitis—urological and gynaecological. At the moment the urological side is always considered first for two reasons:

1 Cystitis, as it stands, belongs to the urinary organs.
2 Cystitis in relation to the kidneys is far more important than cystitis in relation to the uterus in terms of living or dying.

I think there must be very few people who were not given antibiotics on their first experience of the ailment in the last few years. It didn't happen to me in England on my first occasion because I was on honeymoon in Tunisia. The Yugoslav doctor examined me immediately on her treatment couch and between us in pidgin French we just managed to understand each other.

'*Avez-vous le sang?*'
'*Je ne comprends pas, madame.*'
'*Le sang, le sang, comment dit-on en Anglais?*'
She pricked her finger, drew a speck of blood and pointed to it.
'*Ah oui, je comprends, j'ai beaucoup de sang dans l'urine.*'
'*Aha! Madame! vous avez la cystite!*'
And that was it! the soon-to-be-familiar word understandable even in French!

She was very thorough and gave instructions to our accompanying courier to take a specimen to the local hospital in Sousse for testing whilst giving me some pidgin French advice.

'*Pas de sex, pas d'épices, pas d'alcool, pas de natation, madame, pour une semaine*'—no sex, no spicy food, no alcohol, no swimming for one week! Great—what a great holiday let alone a honeymoon! Although I did not understand the words on the laboratory report about my specimen I knew jolly well that the red letters meant something bad and the ordinary black print meant normal.

On top of the verbal advice she prescribed a blue antiseptic pill, some cream and a large penicillin injection to be administered each morning for 5 days by a medical orderly who was on the hotel staff.

It took a good week to recover because I knew nothing about drinking water to flush out the germ—nobody told me. Anyway, that was my first time—each one has a different tale to tell.

My first attack in England arrived three months later. I visited my GP and gave a short account of the Tunisian Tragedy and waited to see what he, an Englishman, would do about it. I was told that probably the Tunisian treatment, although good, had not been of long enough duration to kill the germ entirely, so I was given a month's course of Furadantin. Now anyone on a 5-tablets-a-day dose of this drug knows just how sick you feel.

'Take it with food' I was told at the beginning, 'otherwise you might get nausea.' I stuck it for four days and felt terrible, so I tried, just for the sake of it, taking it without food. This was better and I managed to stay the month's course. A few weeks later, back it came, and more Furadantin was prescribed. Over the next few months and many attacks I was treated with fourteen different types, plus repeat doses, of pills. Sometime later I was given an IVP X-ray and urine tests at a London hospital. On returning for the results I was informed that the kidneys were functioning normally and there were no bacteria present—'Just drink a lot' said the Registrar. 'How much?' said I; 'About 6 pints a day,' he replied. And that was it—'Next patient please'. Not one word of questioning. This by now had taken us up to our first wedding anniversary. Attacks were more frequent—about twice very three weeks and a lot of blood very quickly.

Having been singularly unimpressed with treatment so far by way of the National Health Service, my husband and I decided that, having recovered a little from the early marriage expenses, we might afford a private GP, so we joined BUPA and after a time began private investigations.

My first cystoscopy under general anaesthetic was performed in September 1967, thirteen months after our wedding. Apparently the urethra showed signs of redness and there was also a polyp on the cervix. This was cauterized and I was given a short course of antibiotics and told that was it— all clear. Not a bit of it—back it came with its usual ferocity and regularity.

'Of course, you know,' said my doctor one day, 'that your husband could be infecting you.' 'What with?' I asked. 'Well, there are sorts of infections which can pass between husband and wife. I'll give you both a course of Flagyl which will clear up any trichomonal infections possibly present.'

That night I couldn't bring myself to talk to my husband— fancy, he'd been to blame all through these months. Or had he?—for along came another attack on the last day of the course. For the first time in two years sex was mentioned as possibly being an explanation. I was just about coming to the idea that drinking pints of water during an attack was somewhat helpful, but I felt dreadfully bloated and looked puffy under the eyes at the end of a day having had 14 pints of liquid inside me. I continued on for another eighteen months or so with antibiotics and water, sometimes even injections, until came another IVP X-ray and cystoscopy, both of which were again negative. Four months after, my state of morale was at such a low, having still undergone repeated attacks since that cystoscopy, that my private GP decided to cauterize the urethra—burn away all the infected skin—'you'll never have it again after this'.

Six weeks later he was proved wrong! The story from here I have already told. But to pay ten guineas to hear someone say 'pass water after intercourse' and to have it work is incredible, after all the previous investigations, four and a half years of mismanaged treatment and investigations.

I am not saying useless, because it was undoubtedly worthwhile to know that my kidneys were working, that there was no cancer or tuberculosis in either the renal or sexual organs, but had the GPs told me originally to pass water after intercourse everyone would have profited all round. It takes five seconds to say and costs nothing, as do many of the tips included in the following chapters.

I have discussed at some length my own case history for a couple of reasons. A great many readers will find and recognize many of *its* features in their own experiences. I have always found this aspect of 'in the same boat' extremely comforting and practical. It also shows, as I said, a 'mismanagement', both in the NHS and private sectors, which I feel is a little too frequent.

It is cheaper and quicker to spend time with a patient explaining self-help like strict hygiene, bicarb, liquid intake, etc, etc, than to begin the endless rounds of antibiotics, urine tests, IVPs, cystoscopies and dilations, etc, etc, needlessly.

I intend now to describe some of the aspects of modern investigation and treatment and shall start with antibiotics and urine cultures.

Urinary tract infection is defined as the presence of a specific number of bacteria in the urine. The presence of urinary symptoms is a very unreliable guide to infection and may be associated with other conditions of the urinary tract.

There are two principles which should be followed in the treatment of urinary infection. First, it is necessary to try and isolate the infecting bacteria and this can only be carried out by bacteriological culture of the urine. Second, it is important to determine which of the many available antibiotics or chemotherapeutic substances will be most successful in killing the infecting bacteria.

It is always essential, therefore, to send a specimen of urine for bacteriological examination, even though this may present difficulties for the patient and the doctor. Methods of urine culture are now available which can be carried out in the general practitioner's surgery and these overcome some of the difficulties of urine examination when the hospital laboratory is closed. Where the symptoms are severe, treatment can be started immediately after the urine specimen has been obtained.

The laboratory plays a vital role in the diagnosis of urinary infection but an accurate result can only be obtained when a clean uncontaminated sample of urine is received. In women the specimen should always be collected by the 'mid-stream' method and vulval swabbing should be used. Vulval swabbing involves using gauze swabs moistened with water to clean the vulva and perineal areas and thus prevent organisms from outside the bladder contaminating the urine sample. If contamination should occur the laboratory may not be able to give an accurate result.

The only absolute indications for prescribing treatment for a patient with urinary symptoms are either the presence of a proven urinary infection, or when reasonable steps, i.e. the collection of a urine specimen, have been taken to isolate the infecting bacteria. It is important that treatment should be aimed at killing the bacteria and not only relieving the urinary symptoms.

Chemotherapeutic agents are chemical substances which are used in the treatment of infections and a specific group of these substances called antibiotics were originally derived from living organisms but are now produced synthetically.

The majority of urinary tract infections can be successfully treated with antibiotics taken by mouth (orally) but in a minority of cases it may be important to give injections of antibiotics and in these circumstances it is often necessary to give treatment in hospital.

Although many antibiotics may be suitable for the successful treatment of urinary infection, in many cases one will be most effective in killing the infecting bacteria, and the laboratory can obviously help in directing treatment.

X-RAY INVESTIGATION OF URINARY TRACT

Urinary tract infections are particularly liable to occur in young women—and so is pregnancy. It is necessary to warn patients that, should they suspect that they might be pregnant, their doctor should be informed immediately because any X-ray examination in pregnancy is undesirable except in very special circumstances.

Pyelogram

X-ray investigation of the urinary tract using a dye injected into a vein was first done in 1929 and this has, over the years, become more reliable, safer, and patients experience very few, if any, side-effects. The usual X-ray examination is known as an intravenous pyelogram. This investigation is not necessary in all patients with infection but because it can demonstrate any anatomical abnormality which might form a predisposing cause for repeated infection, it is usually recommended when the condition fails to clear up quickly with simple treatment.

Before having a pyelogram, it is often recommended that the patient should stop drinking for some hours, even from the night before, so that only a little urine is passing through the kidneys at the time of the examination. Usually two pictures are taken at the beginning to show the normal shadows and to demonstrate any stones or radio-opaque abnormalities. An injection is then given into a vein in the arm; this is not painful but occasionally a warm feeling spreads over the whole body just like sitting in a hot bath; but this feeling soon passes off in a few minutes.

The dye, which is opaque to X-rays, then passes through the body and is excreted in the kidneys. As the dye is concentrated in the kidneys a shadow appears which corresponds to the shape and size of the kidneys.

From the kidneys the urine passes through small channels, the calyces, into a collecting funnel, the pelvis, and then down a duct, the ureter, into the bladder. Here the urine remains for a variable period. If there is a pouch (a diverticulum), urine may stagnate in it, or if there is obstruction to the outflow of urine at the neck of the bladder, residual urine may accumulate and be seen on the X-ray.

Obstruction at any point in the collecting system will predispose to infection of the stagnant urine and for this reason patients with recurrent attacks of infection usually have an intravenous pyelogram as a check that the urine is flowing evenly from one part of the urinary system to the next.

The demonstration of any obstruction at the junction of the pelvis with the ureter, or where the ureter joins the bladder, or at the outlet of the bladder may be an indication for surgical intervention, but since the obstruction will then be removed the chances of further attacks of infection are reduced.

Selective Arteriography

The artery to the kidney may be narrowed. In these circumstances a dye can be injected by a long needle inserted into the artery of the thigh. This needle is passed up under television control until it reaches the artery of the kidney. The needle can then be turned directly into the artery and as the dye is injected, the pattern of the arteries can be seen.

Any abnormality such as a cyst or an abscess causes deformity of the arterial pattern. According to the type of deformity various conditions, congenital abnormalities or

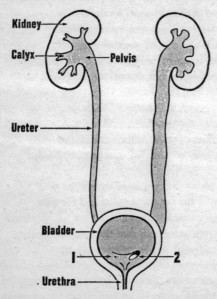

Kidneys
Left: normal pyelogram demonstrating kidney, calyces, pelvis, ureter, bladder and urethra (1). Right: refluxing ureter showing dilated ureteric opening (2) with a distended ureter and clubbing of the calyces. Normal bladder outline

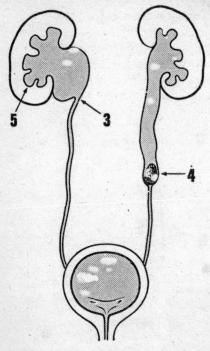

Kidneys
Left: obstruction at the pelvic ureteric junction, distension of the
renal pelvis (3) and blowing out of the calyces (5). Right: stone
impacted in the middle of the ureter, showing an obstructed ureter
above with dilated calyces (4). Normal bladder outline

changes produced by other causes can be diagnosed.

Although this particular injection procedure is not painful
it is very skilled and done under local anaesthetic. It is
therefore usual for the patient to spend the night in hospital.

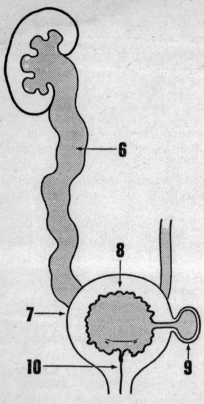

Kidneys
Left: obstructed ureter due to obstruction at the ureterovesical junction (6), thickened bladder wall (7), hypertrophied bladder neck (10). Right: trabeculation of bladder (8), diverticulum of bladder (9)

Nephrotomography

Occasionally it is necessary to get sharper pictures of the kidney—nephrotomography. This is a technique which might be said to focus on different levels of the kidney. Scars in the substance of the kidney or cysts can thus be shown up quite clearly.

Micturating cystogram

Yet another X-ray examination is sometimes called for—a micturating cystogram. Here the radio-opaque dye is inserted by means of a catheter directly into the bladder until it is full. The patient is then asked to pass water, usually standing up, and the way this is done is watched by the radiologist on a closed television screen.

If the urine refluxes back into the kidney it means the valve at the junction of the ureter and the bladder is insufficient and needs repair. If the bladder fails to empty, or if a diverticulum fills up it means there is an obstruction.

As the patient strains, one can see what happens to the bladder neck; if it is wide open it may be the cause of dribbling, or if it descends—as when the uterus prolapses—and doesn't function properly, it may be an indication that the pelvic floor needs further support.

In short, X-ray studies of the urinary tract have made the investigation of recurrent infection an extremely simple, accurate and pain-free procedure, and when some cause is demonstrated the chances of permanent cure by surgery are very good.

CYSTOSCOPY

This, in short, is an examination of the urethra and bladder by an instrument called a cystoscope, and usually has to be done under some form of anaesthetic. The surgeon looks for any

irregularities in these organs and in particular for signs of
bleeding which can simply mean an inflamed, raw, infected
area, or a tumour of some sort. If done by a gynaecologist,
inspection would be made of the vagina and uterus at the
same time, but if the surgeon specializes only in urology then
the examination of the sexual organs may be unlikely.

Together with the results of the IVP the surgeon can assess
all urological aspects of his patient, such as whether the urine
has enough space to pass easily through the urethra. In
America enlarging the urethra, or 'dilating' it, is practised
frequently by urologists and each patient needs it done every
2 to 3 years. Eventually the time gap gets less and less as
attacks become more frequent. Some British specialists regard
it as a 'fashionable' operation with no really proven grounds
for recommending it as a useful treatment. I must say that I
too am sceptical about it. It seems to me that unless there is a
definite blockage or obstruction there is no need to enlarge
what is a perfectly adequate organ for its job as a funnel for
urine.

So much for the major urological investigations and treatments
– now we pass on briefly to genito-urinary and gynaecological
investigations and treatments.

A Genito-Urinary Specialist is one who regards and
assesses the sexual and renal organs together. He does it
mostly for men and is the male substitute for a gynaecologist.

He sees men with prostatitis (infections of the prostate
gland) and men with varying forms of sexually transmitted
diseases. There is a Genito-Urinary Department in all large
hospitals, and if you are told either as a male or female patient
to go for tests you are not thought of as having Venereal
Disease. It is unlawful these days to say that someone has
VD if they only have what is now classed as a sexually
transmitted disease like vaginitis. Babies and children can

have trichomonas simply because their mother did not wash her hands after visiting the toilet. Trichomonas used to be known as belonging to the VD group, but it is not nowadays. The two main groups of VD are gonorrhoea and syphilis—only when tests prove either of these diseases present can you be known as having VD and these come often from promiscuity.

The cystitis sufferer who is really desperate will want to travel all avenues of investigation without qualms—anything to get better, and indeed, in *any* department of medicine the staff are too busy attending to their numbers of patients to bother about assessing whether you are a 'nice' person! If you have even the vaguest suspicion that you may have a discharge whether pink, yellow, white or brown ask your GP for a letter to a genito-urinary department. Many of them nowadays do not even ask for a letter, all they need to treat you is your first telephoned appointment. Ninety-nine times out of a hundred the patient's discharge is due entirely to something else and the department's expert laboratory testing facilities will name the germ very quickly indeed.

I am quite sure that if all patients with discharge or irritation went to one of these departments early on then they would be sorted out painlessly, effectively and swiftly.

The investigations take two forms—a good look-see by the specialist and then various swabs which are sent for immediate culture in the department's laboratory. Treatment for the various types of discharge evolves round pills, some injections, and pessaries and creams according to the cause.

The good gynaecologist has a multitude of causes to prospect. He begins by examining the perineum, looking perhaps for skin that is too tight and splits easily on intercourse; evidence of poor, inefficient hygiene; evidence of haemorrhoids; the presence of itchy red patches either in the pubic hair or just inside the labia majora; any inflammation and where it leads (either up the urethra or vagina). He will not as a rule examine the urethra.

On internal examination of the vagina and cervix he will insert a speculum which slightly props open the walls of the vagina so that he can see as well as feel. The patient either lies on her back or on her side as requested by the individual specialist. There is no pain at all in this process. On sight the gynaecologist looks for evidence of blood; inflammation; abnormal secretions (and if really competent he can tell the difference between the various types of discharge either by its colour, its clarity or its feel). He also looks for dryness; whether the vaginal skin is soft, hard, thin or thick; whether there are any TB spots, lesions or other irregularities.

When he inspects the cervix and uterus he has to apply a little pressure on the outside abdomen to push the uterus downwards for easier examination. Again there is no pain unless there is abnormality. By mostly feeling he can tell

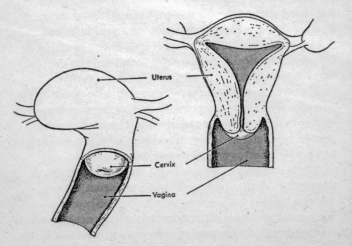

Cervix

whether there are any polyps or growths and whether the uterus is properly positioned. After childbirth a woman's uterus may not have returned to its normal position and can cause pressure on other organs such as the bladder. There are also, as you can see from the small diagram, two cervical openings. One is external and the other the internal mouth. In the canal between, bacteria can rest undisturbed for long periods of time.

Having finished his sight and feel examinations he can then take three swabs—cervical, middle vaginal and, sometimes, perineal. The results will reveal much about the contents of the three areas, but will not, as previously pointed out, show the complete state of hormone balance.

Should anything be felt to be unresolved after all this he can then suggest that the patient be examined under a mild anaesthetic so that the pelvic organs can be better reviewed and also any necessary surgery, like polyp and cyst removal or D & C, be undertaken.

Along these urological and gynaecological exploratory avenues lies the cause of your cystitis, but you must remember that each human body is entirely individual. You must also remember that each doctor is only another human being and although he will do his utmost to get you better he might, through a variety of reasons, just miss your particular cause. This is why the patient is always entitled to a second opinion. With recurrent cystitis the search for the cause must be continuous and ardent for it may even change. It must be undertaken in as detached a manner as possible with full participation in things like note-making during attacks by the patient. It is a game of Snakes and Ladders, and depression must never be allowed to penetrate. Only concentrated, objective thinking by the patient and doctor throughout investigations will reveal the hidden cause.

10 Medical treatment

Well, it must depend, obviously, on the cause. Any doctor giving antibiotics when no infection has been *proved* present will not be helping the patient. Yet antibiotics are given seemingly willy-nilly at the patient's first entrance. Why? Suppose it is eventually proved that there is an obstruction in the kidney–the antibiotics will not cure that! Neither will they cure thrush, trichomonas or prolapsed uterus!

It was almost a year before I was given an IVP–one year I had on solid antibiotic courses with no offer of further investigations. All these investigations should be carried out simultaneously within six months of the established recurrence of attacks. It is only common sense and economy to do so; anything else is false economy; but I'm afraid that this is still the normal order of events. I'll ask again 'Why?'

Population is one answer – too many people to see the doctor each day. He doesn't even have time to read new ideas in the various medical journals and he doesn't seem to take advantage of the GP retraining courses. He is under pressure from drug company salesmen to use their latest and best urinary treatment pills and potions, and after all it is *so* much easier to write a quick prescription than to sit and talk! To give an idea, I received a letter from a GP requesting information about the U and I Club's 'How to Deal with an Attack'. Rather cynically he asked why it had not been printed in the newspaper article which had prompted him to request details. He then said that he had on his books fifteen patients with recurrent cystitis and he was treating them *all* with Urolocosil tablets! ALL of them! Just like sheep-dipping! No thought at all for the individual cause. Those fifteen patients will be permanently on his books and more will be added as the years progress.

Good treatment of cystitis begins, and hopefully ends, in the GP's surgery. For a great many people there is no necessity for any complicated medical treatment, just well-supervised home prevention and management.

Before any medicaments are meted out the patient should receive a list of written instructions for self-help from the GP. It is just as easy as handing out a prescription and may result in the patient's cure. It is far less expensive than drugs and the patient is cheered to think she can help herself in a variety of ways.

If, once the patient is proficient and aware of the importance of all these instructions, attacks are still occurring regularly, then it is certainly necessary to begin the series of investigations as previously described. Only on positive results of a test should treatment begin.

There are nine chemotherapeutic agents commonly used in the treatment of urinary infections. These substances are active against a wide range of bacteria:

Nitrofurantoin

This compound is a chemical substance. It is taken by mouth and should be taken with or after food as it is irritant to the empty stomach in some patients. The most important side-effect is nausea and vomiting but this can usually be overcome either by taking the tablet with food or by reducing the dose.

It is a useful chemotherapeutic agent in the long-term treatment of cystitis and can be prescribed for several months in a single dose taken at night. In recurrent cystitis associated with sexual intercourse a single dose taken within 24 hours of intercourse may prevent an infection. In these two uses it is important to examine samples of urine at intervals to make sure that an asymptomatic infection is not present. Nitrofurantoin can be given to pregnant women but unless the patient is instructed about taking the tablets with or after a meal, vomiting can occur.

Tetracyclines

A large number of compounds are available in this group and, like sulphonamides, there is a variable duration of action and the dose may be taken from one to four times a day. It is effective against most bacteria responsible for urinary tract infection, but there is one species, Proteus mirabilis, which is always resistant. This substance can be safely taken by all patients except young children where bone growth may be retarded and the teeth may acquire a yellow colour. In pregnant women the same changes may occur in the foetus. However, it is very unlikely that these effects would be seen after a short seven-day course of treatment. Other side-effects do occur, particularly intestinal disturbances such as diarrhoea, which is probably due to taking the treatment after meals when the compound will not be completely absorbed resulting in irritation of the intestine. This can be overcome by taking the treatment before meals.

Ampicillin

This substance is one of the penicillin group and was the first member to be effective against the majority of bacteria causing cystitis. In common with all the members of the penicillin family, it can cause a hypersensitivity reaction giving rise to skin rash, and consequently it should not be given to patients who are known to be allergic to penicillin. It is prescribed four times a day and different doses may be used. Occasionally side-effects such as vaginal irritation or discharge may occur. The former will usually resolve without further treatment as it is due to the re-establishment of the normal bacteria in the vagina. However, patients with a persistent vaginal discharge after treatment should consult their doctor as it is possible that this is due to Candida (Monilia or yeast) infection. Gastrointestinal discomfort and diarrhoea may occur and this antibiotic should not be given to patients suffering from glandular fever. It is safe to give to pregnant women.

Cephalexin

This compound is a member of a group of antibiotics called the Cephalosporins. Until recently the available substances in this group could only be given by injection, but cephalexin can be prescribed by mouth. However, it is expensive and it is usually used to treat organisms which would not respond to one of the previous three chemotherapeutic agents. Initially the compound had an unpleasant odour but this has been mainly overcome by purification.

It is prescribed four times a day and can be given to pregnant women, but should be reserved for infections for which other antibiotics would be ineffective and for women allergic to penicillin. Side-effects have been reported and these are mainly nausea, vomiting and diarrhoea, but vaginitis due to a candida or yeast infection can occur.

Sulphonamides

These substances were the earliest antibacterial agents available for the treatment of infection and many different compounds are used. Two main groups occur, first those that are absorbed when given by mouth and will be effective in the treatment of urinary tract infection and second, those that are not absorbed into the body and can only be used for the treatment of intestinal infections.

The original sulphonamides had a short action and treatment was given every six hours, but recently sulphonamides with a longer action have been introduced and dosage may be either once a day or, with the very long-acting compounds, only a single dose is required for the complete course of treatment. The new sulphonamides are safe substances and are effective against the majority occurring in 'simple' (uncomplicated) urinary tract infections. The incidence of side-effects is low, but skin rashes, nausea and very occasionally vomiting can occur. Sulphonamides can be safely prescribed in pregnancy up to the thirty-sixth week.

Nalidixic acid

This is another chemical substance like nitrofurantoin which is produced synthetically. Although the original compound produced many bizarre side-effects, subsequently purification has eliminated these and few reactions occur. It is given three or four times a day. Although no untoward reactions have been reported, it should probably not be used in the early stages of pregnancy.

Trimethoprin and sulphamethoxazole

This substance which is a combination of a sulphonamide with a long-action and a chemical compound has recently been introduced.

Trimethoprin has few side-effects, and those reactions which occur in patients on treatment are due to the sulphonamide component and can be skin rashes or nausea. It is prescribed twice a day and is one of the few chemotherapeutic agents that are available in the form of a suspension for adults. The tablets are large and difficult to

swallow for some patients. It is advisable not to give this
substance to pregnant women.

Penicillin

This is one of the earliest antibiotics discovered and it still
has the greatest activity of all chemotherapeutic substances
against sensitive bacteria. Unfortunately, many of the
organisms causing urinary tract infections are resistant, but
it is excreted in large amounts in the urine and is a very useful
treatment in some infections. It should not be given to patients
known to be allergic and even so skin rashes may occur due to
the presence of undiagnosed or unknown allergy.

Amoxycillin

This substance is also a member of the Penicillin group and is
effective against the same strains of bacteria as Ampicillin.
However, it is better absorbed into the body and may be very
effective in the treatment of more resistant bacteriuria.
Side-effects are similar to Ampicillin although
gastrointestinal symptoms are seen less frequently. Allergy
to Penicillin is an absolute contraindication to its use. It is
safe to use in pregnancy.

This description of the antibiotics commonly used in the
treatment of urinary tract infection has purposely not indicated
which substances are best or what dose should be given and
for how long, as it is impossible to generalize for every
infection.

Treatment must primarily depend on the nature of the
infecting bacteria and sensitivity to a wide range of antibiotics.
Secondly, the dose will depend on the clinical nature of the
infection and the past clinical history of the individual patient.
The length of treatment will also be variable, as in some
infections a short course using a large dose is indicated

whereas in others it may be necessary to give a small dose of an antibiotic for a course lasting several weeks or months.

Lastly, where two antibiotics are equally effective it is wise in economic terms to prescribe the cheaper.

It is essential, therefore, to try and isolate the infecting organism in urinary tract infection and not to prescribe treatment blindly. Although it may necessitate delaying treatment for at least twenty-four hours the benefits of knowing the nature of the infecting bacteria and the most effective treatment are invaluable.

After these antibiotics have been taken, it would be advisable to check for thrush. If thrush is found, various treatments can be tried:

Nystan pills and Nystatin pessaries used in conjunction with one another.
Sporastacin vaginal cream with an applicator.
Candeptin vaginal ointment with an applicator.
Gentian Violet solution swabbed high into the vagina.
Fungilin mouth lozenges, because thrush can also be present on the tongue.

Again, no distinction is made here between them but it is important that all creams and pessaries be placed high in the vagina. It is advisable to insert two pessaries, not to sit in the bathwater, and to wear a small pad for the duration of the treatment.

Any person being treated with antibiotics for any medical reason must be regarded as a potential thrush victim and appropriate preventive treatment prescribed before it takes a hold.

Once thrush has been eradicated, no more antibiotics should be administered for cystitis except doses of three days' duration only with several months between each course. If the specialist does insist on antibiotics then a constant watch must be kept for thrush.

It may be that this was the cause anyway, so one waits with bated breath for another recurrence of cystitis.

If and when it does recur, all previously described investigations must begin. Let us take a few of the more obvious causes that may be found during tests and assessments.

Suppose an IVP X-ray shows a kidney stone lodged in the ureter. Preliminary treatment is excessive water intake to try to flush the stone down and out. If this fails, attempts are made to remove it surgically.

Treatment for trichomoniasis

A sexually transmitted disease, *trichomoniasis* responds to Flagyl tablets and it is wise to give courses of between one and two weeks' duration to husband and wife at the same time.

Treatment for refluxing ureter

This occurs mostly in children when the urine is squirted back up the ureter by a faulty valve mechanism. Treatment is generally by semi-permanent antibiotics to reduce and control infection until general muscle development at the age of eight might resolve the problem by strengthening the weak valve. If this does not occur then surgery is undertaken to repair or replace the valve or even to divert the urine flow to the other ureter. But it is a major operation and only performed when all other treatment has failed (diagram in Chapter 9).

Treatment for hormone imbalance

When once assessed by even a competent gynaecologist, it can still take a little while to find out what sort of dosage is best for each patient. Treatment mainly consists of oestrogen either in cream for local application or taken as a pill, orally, or maybe by injection or implant. Sometimes progestogen is given and sometimes a combination of both of these hormones. A close watch must be kept on the patient who should also observe her feelings if possible and report any adverse effects. I always try to explain these drugs like this: The body needs a great many ingredients to keep it happy and healthy, like proteins, iron, calcium, etc. Hormones are just another ingredient. If you have too few you won't work so well! The 'booster' treatment can last anything from one month to several years depending on the severity of symptoms and any female age group between fifteen and sixty-five years can be susceptible to stress changes in their hormone balance. Few women get off scot-free in the menopause from all the usual menopausal symptoms, i.e. hot flushes and odd spells of feeling off-colour; likewise women undergoing a hysterectomy. But when symptoms including urinary problems are severe then hormone boosters will improve the situation and make life a little more bearable. Oddly enough, female hormones help a lot in the case of male prostate cancer. They shrivel up the carcinoma and open up the water passage so that urine can flow properly.

Bladder wash-outs

A catheter is gently inserted into the urethra and up into the bladder. Any urine present is drawn off or squeezed out and the bladder is then filled with any one of a variety of solutions from simple sterile water right through to a strongish antiseptic solution. This treatment is used mostly for bladder encrustation or for giving comfort to carcinoma patients. Obviously its use depends on how highly it is rated by any particular surgeon, and it should never be performed by the patient. Although no anaesthetic is needed, conditions of sterility are vital and the bed needs to be well protected.

Treatment for kidney infection
It depends on keeping the kidneys well washed out, plus administration of the drug to which the cultured bacteria are sensitive. If infection is progressive and prolonged then there is a very real chance of renal failure. Dialysis—cleansing the blood by passing it through a kidney machine—may be recommended and later still the removal of one or both kidneys. A patient with one kidney lives quite a full life and indeed kidney transplants are now a part of our modern medical life.

Repairs of prolapsed uterus
Mostly it means surgery in terms of treatment. The uterus is repositioned and the lax vaginal tissues repaired. It is a matter of removing the pressure from the bladder wall and strengthening those muscles in the pelvis allowed to sag following childbirth.

Hysterectomy
Hysterectomy is never performed solely for cystitis, but if there is some major disorder of the uterus which might happen to have cystitis as one of its effects then obviously the patient will benefit from the removal of the uterus.

Cauterization
This is mostly used to remove chronic infected tissue particularly in the urethra and cervix. Generally performed under an anaesthetic, an electrically heated metal rod burns away affected tissues. It is said to be a favourite Japanese remedy. However, its success is never guaranteed.

Dilatation
This is simply enlargement of the cervix or urethra by inserting metal rods one by one until the stretching process is

complete. Sometimes done without an anaesthetic to the urethra, it can be painful.

There, then, are summaries of some of the main medical or surgical treatment processes at present in use for the relief of bladder ailments and some associated conditions. Variations occur on these themes dependent upon the surgeon's likes and dislikes and the patient's personal problem. All these treatments work their best when supported by the aware and educated patient in her home, and it is to this cooperational end that we approach the final chapter.

11 Self-help

The overriding object of this book is that you, the patient, can be given some much-desired information and education on the subject of cystitis. I have explained as much as I feel can be understood and assimilated by the average person about the technicalities which lurk in the background of each attack.

Now I am going to teach you ways in which to help yourself. All our information is drawn from other patients' experiences, medically reviewed and then re-presented as expertly as possible so that you are receiving the most modern advice available.

We shall sub-divide the chapter into two headings, the first of which is Prevention.

PREVENTION

As we know, urinary infections can either ascend from the perineum or descend from the bloodstream and kidneys.

Ascending infections can be assumed when symptoms of the first attack seem to start at the urethral opening and over the first hour or so are felt to travel upwards and into the bladder.

Descending infections may produce a variety of symptoms which can also be symptomatic of other ailments totally unrelated, i.e. backache, pains in the abdomen, general tiredness and mild bladder disturbance.

Let us take the ascending type first because this can, in the main, be prevented by the patient.

Hygiene
I can hear you all shouting 'I bath every day'. Unfortunately this is not enough. Some people have a lot more E-coli in their bowels than others and the perineum, therefore, needs washing more frequently. Keep a special isolated flannel for yourself and wash the area each morning, evening and always after passing a stool. Use just a little pure soap and warm water and then rinse and dry thoroughly. Make sure that no soap is left to irritate. Never use powder, cream, antiseptic, antibiotic cream or vaginal deodorants—only warm or cool water. A bidet is ideal and even more thorough than a flannel. The best one seems to be that which has a small, controllable fountain of water in the middle of the bidet so that only fresh water touches the skin, no hand contact being needed.

Speaking of hands, I'm sure there is little necessity to explain that hands carry germs and must be washed before they attempt to cleanse the genitalia.

Underwear: pants and knickers must be changed every day. Preferably made of cotton, they should be boiled regularly and aired well. Much has been said about the part which nylon tights and girdles play in urinary infections. Nylon materials do not allow air to circulate; they form a barrier, and that is one of the reasons why they are never worn in hot countries. Heat makes the body perspire and become clammy. The same is true of the perineum. It feels better when cool—not cold—and germs find it more difficult to breed when the skin is dry.

It could be rather risky to wear tights *and* a panty girdle together. If the weather is hot and you must wear tights because your dress is short, then try to find some with a

cotton gusset or make a point of washing at the first opportunity on your return home. Vaginal thrush is also more
active in hot weather so try whenever possible to go without
tights and girdle. A belt and stockings will give the same
support but allow the perineum to remain as fresh as possible.
I expect you will work something out for yourselves.

As far as washing underwear is concerned, make sure that,
whatever the washing powder, you rinse and rinse again
until the rinsing water is perfectly clear. Avoid bleaches or
strong powders.

Remember that whatever bacteria are on your underwear
will shortly be on your skin and vice versa!

Douching

In recent years this seems to have fallen out of fashion.

But why should the vagina be expected to go without a
good wash? The urethra, next door, gets cleaned and flushed
through several times a day even though it has fewer outside
influences. The vagina, unless douched out, has all sorts of
natural secretions which can become stale and create breeding
grounds for germs. On top of this the sexually active female
using any other form of contraceptive except her partner's
sheath has lubricants, foams, jellies, pessaries, and semen to
store. The effect of all these liquids in an un-douched vagina
can be rather unwholesome. Once a week douching, using
cool water, will clear out all the stale secretions, and if you
have never used one you will immediately notice how much
cleaner and nicer you feel.

Internal tampons are best not used when cystitis is a
problem. The cotton wool may contain various additives
which could harm the sensitive vagina—they are also very
drying.

Acid or alkaline?

This question is often asked, and so often left improperly answered. The normal urine is moderately acidic and if E-coli finds its way into this urine either in the urethra or bladder then it will start to breed. Once this state of affairs has arisen and an attack is imminent then the urine must be made alkaline to prevent any further progress by the germ.

To make the urine highly acidic means drinking nothing but pure fruit juices, and not very many anyway. You will pass very little water and what you do pass will be uncomfortable, possibly even burning badly if you are having an actual attack. The kidneys are not flushed through, neither are the bladder and the urethra, and the whole process is somewhat arduous with no real assurance that the kidneys are remaining unconnected with the ascending infection. There are, however, some drugs which work best in an acid urine, but on this your doctor must give individual advice.

To make the urine alkaline is far easier, although it must be pointed out that anyone suffering from heart trouble must first ask permission from their doctor before taking bicarbonate of soda. One teaspoon of bicarbonate may be taken twice a day when the urine becomes too acid and also when an attack is starting. It tastes best when disguised with orange or lemon squash.

The surest way of discovering whether your urine is acid or normal is to buy red litmus papers costing between 5p and 10p a packet. Dip one in your urine whenever it burns; if the paper remains pink or red then the urine is acid and you may take one teaspoon of bicarbonate until the paper turns into tones of blue.

Alcohol

One word sums up this section: 'Never'. Well, almost never!

Alcohol is a trigger factor to any patient with a sensitive bladder because it causes dehydration and changes the urine to a high acidity level. Little urine is then excreted by the kidneys and consequently the important diluted urine flow is absent. The bladder becomes dry and sore and what little urine there is, burns.

This action is not quite as severe when long alcoholic drinks are taken. Two or three pints of beer or Guinness, for instance, contain quite a lot of ordinary water and so long as a couple of glasses of bland liquid are drunk as a follow-up there is no reason to stop imbibing occasionally!

Shorts—of whisky, gin, vodka, etc, are fatal! Never, ever touch these if you are prone to cystitis.

Liqueurs—none of these, either, because the spirit proof is also very high.

Champagne—well it seems a bit too saintly to resist just one glass—so have one glassful, make it last and when it's finished go and drink some orange squash and be grateful that you have not put your bladder in an awkward spot!

Wine—very difficult to take a firm stand because most of us enjoy a glass or two of wine. If you know you are going to drink some wine with your meal, drink half a pint of something bland beforehand and again *after* the meal. The best type of wine is a light German Hock. The French, true gastronomers all, regard such wine rather cynically as mere lemonade! Never mind, it tastes delicious and doesn't do much harm to your bladder!

Red wine is really very difficult but if you limit yourself to one glass and do the same thing of sandwiching it between two half-pints of bland liquids, or diluting it with water, then you are considerably reducing its alcoholic effect.

Aperitifs—again difficult because they also contain high spirit levels. You should be thinking in terms of a long drink which will last you whilst everyone else gets through two or three rounds of shorts.

Try the following:
Double tomato juice with half-measure dry sherry and no Worcestershire sauce.
Single Martini, Dubonnet or Cinzano in a large glass filled up with either water, soda water or tonic water and ice.

It's amazing what you can make yourself get used to!

Hexachlorophene

Although mentioned in the chapter headed 'Children' this ingredient of many toiletries is sufficiently problematical to warrant another mention. The Government has now banned its use in all children's toiletries, but nothing has been done about withdrawing it from adult products. Before you buy any soap, powder, deodorant or shampoo look at the named contents. Do not buy any that contain Hexachlorophene or Chlorohexaphene. Unfortunately some manufacturers seem to throw a little in and not name its presence, so only use tried and tested soaps known for their purity.

Descending infections really cannot be prevented by the patient—the only thing to do is to keep 6 to 8 pints of liquid going through the kidneys each day to wash away as many bacteria as possible. Your doctor may be able to give further ideas because only he has full knowledge of your medical history.

Sexual causes

Apart from enabling man and woman to breed children, sexual intercourse may also enable two sets of germs to breed and multiply.

Relating urinary problems to intercourse can be done fairly accurately by counting back from the attack 1 night and 1 day *or* 1 night, 1 day and 1 more night.

If it is the former, then 'bruising and trauma' are likely to be the only cause—not a germ, at least not to start with; lax hygiene may later bring about a bacterial infection sited on the bruised or inflamed area. This is the main cause of honeymoon cystitis and holiday cystitis. One cannot expect the delicate tissues of the vagina to withstand intercourse more than once a day; preferably there should be a gap of two days for the recurrent sufferer. KY Jelly by Johnson & Johnson will lessen the risk of bruising. I wonder how many people go and have a long soak in a hot bath after intercourse? This sometimes does quite a lot of harm, firstly because the vagina is not really being washed, and secondly the hot water soaking into slightly swollen vaginal and urethral orifices will prolong the swellings. If you accidentally bruise some other part of your body you make sure the skin is not broken—if it is, you wash it gently and keep it clean. Do not use any antiseptic solution on the genitalia, only cold water or sterile swabs of cotton wool. You should also make sure that you do not bump the bruise again—walking has this effect on reddened and swollen genitalia, so rest if possible.

An old-fashioned but very soothing aid for bruising is witchhazel and it can also take away those 'twinges' of early soreness on the perineum. This lotion helps a lot of people, but again it rests largely with the individual.

If you relate your urinary symptoms back 1 night, 1 day and 1 more night, or 36 hours, it is because germs have had time to multiply. These germs can come from the male or female. Swabs of the vagina will disclose any germs there and an immediate urine culture will reveal the germ causing the cystitis in the urethra and bladder. It will save a lot of time and suffering if the male also has some tests. If he is uncircumcised and finds difficulty in cleansing the foreskin it is only common sense to use the condom as a form of contraceptive. Watch for any soreness stemming from lubricants, creams, foams, etc, and experiment until you find a satisfactory sex routine that does not result in soreness and pain.

If, however, your hygiene and follow-up routine is really efficient then infection from E-coli has little chance to begin. Unusual vaginal discharges must be reported as they will probably 'ping-pong' between the sexual partners so no amount of washing will help here.

There is, however, one superb and vital piece of self-help in the incidence of cystitis related to intercourse. It cost me ten guineas in a Harley Street consulting room and saved my marriage.

It is: Always pass an effective amount of urine within fifteen minutes of intercourse ending, and then wash. This is because E-coli, as we know, multiply by thousands every 12·5 minutes. If you flush out any stray germs, which have been thrust into the bladder during intercourse, by passing water, infection cannot commence, so nature comes to our aid without any need of manmade pills.

Always work with nature not against her. Just what is the good of pouring antibiotics into the bladder when all the poor thing needs is a little understanding help in order to work happily and painlessly.

Holidays
Take the bathroom cabinet *with* you! You may even find your doctor amenable to providing you with a holiday prescription of say 12 antibiotic capsules in case all that you try in the way of management of an attack fails completely. My mail order company can supply many of the

products mentioned in this chapter in reasonable quantities.
Ask for our latest catalogue by sending a stamped, addressed
envelope to Angela Kilmartin Mail Order, 22 Gerrard Road,
London N1.

Make a list:

Bicarbonate of soda—2 packets
Special flannels—2 or 3
Pure soap
Douche
12 antibiotic capsules
KY Jelly—1 tube
Cottonwool swabs
Water sterilizing pills—1 packet
Sporastacin (for thrush if you are prone in hot weather)—
    1 tube
A bottle of Dr J. Collis Browne's Chlorodyne (to keep the
bowels working slowly!)
Hot water bottles—2 (I'll tell you why later)

Swimming is allowed providing you take enough bathing
suits. Never sit in a damp or wet suit in the sun—the rest of the
body warms up but the abdomen, kidneys and urethra stay
cold. Once out of the water, be it fresh, sea or pool water,
go up to your bedroom and change. Pass any urine
accumulated in the bladder and then wash either on the bidet
or with a special flannel. Rinse off exceptionally well, getting
rid, in the process, of salt or chlorine deposits. This is
important because, if left, these granules can chafe away for
hours, eventually making you very sore. What is more, you
never quite know what else is in the water! So, if in doubt,
wash it out!

If the holiday heat is high then be a little daring in your
longer dresses and go without underwear. Cooler air can

then circulate, lessening the risk of thrush starting up in the perspiration droplets.

Keep some still or fizzy bottled water in your bathroom. Have a good swig at it each morning before breakfast if you are abroad because it gives the kidneys a good start to the day by clearing out any bacterial residue. It is important for the urinary patient to drink a lot of water in the heat. The flushing and washing through process must be kept up otherwise you will become dehydrated, and mind you obey the alcohol rules even though it is holiday time.

We all obviously have to travel to get to our holiday resort. Please don't economize by taking the coach; the stops are infrequent and the result is a frustrated, tearful holiday-maker. Rather go by train or plane where there are toilet facilities, and then book in at a cheaper hotel if you need to economize. Urinary patients really shouldn't have touring holidays either unless towing their own caravan and toilet!

If you have decided to go to Greenland take some long woollen combinations!

If the worst comes to the worst when abroad you'll find your foreign pocket dictionary handy—I learnt my lesson on holiday when I couldn't remember the French for 'blood'!

Above all, have a rest! See if Grandma or Great Aunt can have the children for a week and then go anywhere where you can put your feet up. A relaxed and cheerful mind just doesn't go with aching feet! You'll therefore fight your problems more fiercely and courageously if your body and soul are held together by good holidays!

MANAGEMENT

If all your preventive measures fail and the cause of your attacks has not been discovered either by you or your

doctors then you need to have a special routine at your
fingertips to manage each attack of cystitis.

The time at which the attack begins can also be helpful in
relating the attack to a particular area of causes. For instance
when it begins during the day and intercourse has not taken
place in the previous 36 hours then one can assume that the
cause is unrelated to sex—though not entirely, as I have
previously shown, because there are any number of vaginal
conditions to contend with. Intercourse is mostly nocturnal
and any related attack due to infection will almost certainly
start 36 hours later between the hours of 2am and 10am.
Mine mostly used to begin around three or four o'clock.

Never turn over in bed and try to forget it! Those early
'twinges' and sensations exist as a helpful warning and you
deserve everything you get if you ignore them. It will not
go away and will certainly get much worse.

So get up and set your mind to treating yourself in as
practical a way as possible. It won't help to cry and moan;
it will be better if you concentrate on becoming a nurse for
the next three hours. Through your own practical treatment
and management you will know that you can control the
pain and the infection and this alone will distract your
depressive thoughts. There is no doubt that recurrent attacks
are horribly depressive. It does no good to beat your hands
on the nearest wall and floor or to sit for ages in the bathroom
crying.

Having once put all the treatment in hand you have odd
minutes between visiting the bathroom to write down any
clues as to the cause of the attack, for your doctor. Having
read the book this far you should know a little about what to
look for. When you have exhaustively searched your mind
and put your discoveries in writing you will need further
mental distractions. Someone I know does crosswords; others

read books, newspapers, play Patience or sew tapestry, and I used to start my washing when the pain and frequency lessened towards the end of the three hours. On a summer morning it can be marvellous hanging out the shirts at six o'clock! The birds are singing and the sun filters through our plane tree and both experiences are made more poignant by the smell of dewy earth, roses and honeysuckle–really lovely! As I said, you must lift your mind above the physical pain or life will really take a tumble.

It takes three hours to alleviate an attack of cystitis using the following method. It is designed to prevent *you* reaching desperation and the *infection* from reaching the ureters and kidneys. The method can be commenced anywhere that is fairly private with a comfy chair or bed, a lavatory and a handbasin. It works far more effectively and quickly than any other method and needs no antibiotics or medicines to help.

How to deal with an attack of cystitis
Pass a specimen into a clean, closed container so that your GP may culture the germ, and then:

Get up and go to your kitchen. Put the kettle on for two hot water bottles. Take from your cupboard a large water jug and glass.

Immediately drink one pint of cold water and let your stomach settle for a while.

Find the bicarbonate of soda and, when the kettle has boiled and the hot water bottles are filled, drink $\frac{1}{4}$ of a glass of orange squash mixed with 1 teaspoon of bicarbonate. This is to be done three times in the next three hours. (Again, remember that heart patients must discuss the bicarbonate with their specialist.)

Take two tablets of a mild painkiller, perhaps either Disprin or Paracetamol.

Fill the water jug and glass with bland liquid.

Once each hour have a strong black coffee. Coffee is a diuretic and a bladder irritant. It is helpful now because we want the bladder nerve fibres to work overtime in helping to pass water, otherwise coffee should not be drunk at all by bladder patients.

Before you go back to bed or to your chair with your jug and glass have another half pint of liquid. Barley waters make life a little easier.

Put one hot water bottle on your back and the other high up between the legs resting if possible between the labia. Wrap a towel round this bottle so that it doesn't burn but only heats.

Every time you pass water go and wash the perineum gently. Dab it dry, don't rub it!

You have now given yourself a good fighting start, and you then carry on drinking half a pint of liquid every 20 minutes making sure that you are also passing large amounts. The coffee helps this action but if your doctor would let you keep a few diuretic pills in the house for this reason it will help the flushing process to take two tablets right at the beginning. These tablets must not be taken unless prescribed by your doctor.

If the attack worsens a little in the first half-hour it is only because the treatment has not yet reached the urethra, so don't worry, just keep pouring the liquid down.

This, then, is your last-ditch stand. When the method is performed correctly you need no longer fear an attack, you will be back at work in a much shorter time than you have ever been previously.

Here ends our chapter on Self-help. It has been of necessity a long chapter and I hope that you have learnt from it and will use it whenever necessary. Keep reading it—you just might have missed something out!

Summary

Cystitis is a very complex subject and some aspects of it have puzzled and still are puzzling medical minds. We, the patients, have at last seen ways of helping our doctors to help us and this combined action may lead us all a little further along the road of knowledge.

This is the first book on the subject written by a patient; possibly others will follow. Until that time this book will represent hope and a new way of living for countless thousands of people. For myself it is the culmination of victory over my own cystitis problems because there were four-and-a-half years in my twenties when tears and pain were very frequent occurrences. I shall be prone to cystitis all my life but I know a lot about it now and I know my own personal causes; therefore I can prevent and manage it. There will be rare future attacks which may possibly not come within my area of knowledge but my doctor may well know the answer and with his cooperation and mine we will triumph. Your attitude must be the same.

Glossary of terms

ANAEMIA low level of iron in the blood.

ARTERY blood vessel carrying blood *from* the heart.

BACTERIA germs.

CATHETERIZATION insertion of small tube to withdraw urine from the bladder.

CAUTERIZATION burning away of infected skin.

CERVIX neck of the womb.

CYSTOSCOPY operation for investigation of the bladder.

DIABETES illness caused by excess sugar in the bloodstream.

DIALYSIS artificial cleansing of blood by machine.

DILATATION enlargement of cervix or urethra by insertion of rods.

DISTAL URETHRAL STENOSIS condition of the urethra during menopause or old age.

DIVERTICULUM small false bladder growth.

E-COLI Escherichia Coli, natural bacterial inhabitants of the bowel.

ENURESIS childhood or adult bed-wetting.

EPITHELIUM skin.

FLORA AND FAUNA natural organisms populating any part of the body.

FORESKIN superfluous skin on the penis.

FUNGUS growth of detrimental organisms.

GONADOTROPHIN hormone involved in ovulation.

HEXACHLOROPHENE an antiseptic.

HORMONE a chemical messenger carrying instructions from glands to organs.

HORMONE IMBALANCE incorrect hormone balance.

HYSTERECTOMY removal of all or part of the female sexual organs.

INTRAVENOUS into the vein (injections).

IVP intravenous pyelogram—kidney X-rays.

MENOPAUSE natural process involving termination of menstruation.

MICTURITION act of passing urine.

MSU mid-stream urine specimen.

OESTROGEN hormone involved in ovulation.

ORIFICE opening.

OVULATION release of unfertilized female egg from the ovaries.

PERINEUM base of the body's trunk containing excretal orifices.

PITUITARY GLAND chief sexual gland of the brain responsible for most hormone activity.

PROGESTOGEN hormone involved in ovulation.

PROLAPSE displaced organ.

PROSTATE GLAND male sexual gland through which passes the male urethra.

PYELITIS kidney disease.

RECTUM tube for passage of stools.

REFLUX urine flow in the wrong direction.

RENAL SCARRING scarring of the kidney by constant disease.

SPHINCTER VALVE valve attached to the sphincter muscles controlling output of urine.

TRICHOMONAS sexually transmitted disease.

URETERS tubes carrying urine from the kidneys.

URETHRA tube carrying urine from the bladder.

URETHRAL SYNDROME medically unaccountable symptoms of urinary infection.

UTERUS womb.

VAGINA birth canal.

VAGINAL THRUSH milky discharge from the vagina.

VEIN blood vessel carrying blood *to* the heart.

Index

Acidity, 106
Alcohol, 107–8
Alkalinity, 106
Allergies, 73, 97
Amoxycillin, 97
Ampicillin, 94–5
Anaemia, 60–61
Antibiotics, 17, 22–3, 35, 79, 92
Antibodies, 27

Barley Water, 45, 115
Bicarbonate of soda, 50, 114
Bladder, 66–8
  wash-out, 100
Blood, 65, 77, 90
Bruising, 20–22, 109

Candeptin, 98
Catheterization, 31, 68
Causes of cystitis
  gynaecological, 20
  renal, 28–31
  sexual, 20–23, 108–9
Cauterization, 10, 101
Cephalexin, 95
Cervix, 90–91
Childbirth, 27, 91
Children, 37, 73–6
Contraception, 25

Cystitis
  causes of, 20–23, 28–31,
    108–9
  depression, 12
  management of, 112–15
  prevention of, 103–12
  recurrent, 12
  symptoms of, 16
Cystoscopy, 13, 15, 79, 87–8

Depression, 12, 34, 40, 62
Diabetes, 30
Dilatation, 101–2
Discharges, 89
Diverticulum, 30–31
Douching, 105

E-coli, 21–2
Enuresis, 74–6

Fungilin, 98

Genito-urinary specialists, 88
Gentian violet, 98

Herpes, 31
Hexachlorophene, 73–4, 108
Holidays, 33–4, 110–11
Honeymoon, 20–21, 33–5, 40

Hormones, 23–5
  imbalance, 23–5, 61–4
  stress, 72
  testing for, 62
  treatment for, 99–100
Hygiene, 35, 47–8, 104–5
Hysterectomy, 101

Incontinence, 11
Intercourse, 11
Intravenous pyelogram (IVP),
  78, 83–4
Iron injections, 60

Kidneys, 65–6
  failure of, 17
  infection of, 101
  stones, 31
  transplant, 69
  treatment for, 101

Lubricant, 26, 109

Marriage, 33–5
Menopause, 63, 100

Nalidixic acid, 96
Nerve fibres, 67–9
Nitrofurantoin, 93–4
Nystan, 98
Nystatin, 98

Orifices
  rectal, 20
  urethral, 20
  vaginal, 20

Penicillin, 97
Perineum, architecture of, 20
Pregnancy, 28
Prolapse, 87
  uterus, 28, 87
Prostatitis, 50–51
Psychiatric help, 12
Pyelitis, 17
Pyelogram, 78, 83–4

Renal
  failure, 17, 69
  mechanism, 65
  organs, 65–6
  surgery, 13

Self-help, 113–15
Sexual
  activity, 20–23
  organs, 59–63
Soap, 48
Sphincter, 66–7
Spinal cord, 67
Sporastacin, 98
Stress, 24, 70–72
Sulphamethoxazole, 96–7
Sulphonamides, 95–6
Swabs, vaginal, 23, 98

Tetracyclines, 94
Thrush, 105
  treatment of, 98–9
Tranquillizers, 12
Trichomonas, 22, 79
Trichomoniasis, 99
Trimethoprin, 96–7

U and I Club
  aim, 36
  founded, 9
  set of rules, 18
  survey, 12–13
Underwear, 104–5
Ureter
  mechanics of, 66
  reflux, 30, 99
Urethra, 67
  bruising of, 109
  cauterization, 10, 101
Urethral syndrome, 71
Urinary infection, research, 9
Urine, 10, 39, 66
  specimens, 39, 77, 114

Uterus, 27, 90
  prolapsed, 28, 87

Vagina, 62
Vaginal
  epithelium, 12
  thrush, 22
VD, 33, 88–9
Vulval swabbing, 81

Witchhazel, 48, 109

X-rays, 78, 82–8
  micturating cystogram, 87
  nephrotomography, 87
  pyelogram, 82–3
  selective arteriography, 84–5

STRESS: THE MODERN SICKNESS 60p
Peter Blythe

Why is stress an ever-increasing problem?

How does the mind convert stress into physical illness?

What can be done to combat stress-disease?

These and many other vital questions are discussed by Peter Blythe, a practising psychotherapist and consultant hypnotist, who examines every aspect of normal living and shows how the build-up of anxiety-stress-tension plays a determining part in a variety of illnesses including

Hypertension (high blood pressure)   Diabetes mellitus
Coronary thrombosis   Skin disorders
Migraine   Rheumatoid arthritis
Hay fever   Menstrual difficulties
Asthma   Peptic ulcers

'Fascinating . . . to me his conclusions make a lot of sense. And I would warmly recommend that anyone who feels unwell for no reason that the doctor can find, anyone who has received a doctor's diagnosis of "nerves", anyone who is facing marital or personal difficulties which are preventing good health or a full and happy life could not do better than face facts and ask themselves if stress might not be the root of the trouble'

NURSE WILLIAMS, WOMAN MAGAZINE

THE DOCTOR'S QUICK
WEIGHT LOSS DIET 30p
Irwin Maxwell MD and Samm Sinclair Baker

Medically proved – lose 5 to 15 pounds a week with this safe, spectacular new diet breakthrough by a practising physician who has personally helped 10,000 patients to lose excess weight easily, quickly and safely.

Vital truths about effective dieting smash the common misconception that slowly cutting down on food is the only 'proper' way to reduce.

Over 60 quick reducing diets to fit every problem and taste
The answers to dieters' common complaints – and excuses
The all-important principles of dieting psychology
How to stay slim once the weight has been lost

This book contains no way-out theories or strange concoctions. Its instructions are simple to understand, easy to follow – and have been proved dramatically effective by the eminent and experienced doctor who wrote this highly acclaimed work.

PREGNANCY £1·50
Gordon Bourne FRCS FRCOG

'The most authoritative and comprehensive guide to pregnancy, labour and motherhood'
VOGUE

Having a child can be one of the most exciting and fulfilling experiences in a woman's life, provided she has the confidence that comes from knowing exactly what pregnancy involves.

This comprehensive guide is written by Dr Gordon Bourne, Consultant Obstetrician and Gynaecologist to one of London's leading teaching hospitals. It provides full information, guidance and reassurance on all aspects of pregnancy and childbirth. An indispensable aid to the expectant mother, it will also be of great interest and use to her husband and family.

'Sets out in a clear, factual and reassuring way every possible aspect of pregnancy . . . I would recommend this book to anyone who can buy or borrow a copy'
MARRIAGE GUIDANCE